navel ⟨ ° ⟩ gazing

Jennifer Matesa

PHOTOGRAPHS BY CHARLEE BRODSKY

THREE RIVERS PRESS · NEW YORK

navel (°) gazing

The Days and Nights of a Mother in the Making

Published by Three Rivers Press, New York, New York.

Member of the Crown Publishing Group.

Random House, Inc. New York, Toronto, London, Sydney, Auckland

www.randomhouse.com

THREE RIVERS PRESS is a registered trademark and the Three Rivers Press
colophon is a trademark of Random House, Inc.

Printed in the United States of America

Design by Elina D. Nudelman

Library of Congress Cataloging-in-Publication Data

Matesa, Jennifer.
Navel-gazing : the days and nights of a mother in the making
by Jennifer Matesa.
Includes bibliographical references.
pbk.
1. Matesa, Jennifer. 2. Pregnant women—Biography. 3. Pregnancy—
Psychological aspects. 4. Childbirth—Psychological aspects. I. Title.
RG525 .M355 2001
618.2'4'092—dc21
B   2001023948

ISBN 0-609-80787-0

10 9 8 7 6 5 4 3 2 1

First Edition

*f*or Nick and Jonathan,
my men,

and in memory of Mary Matesa,
my mother

Also for Mark, Gillian, and Allyn

Contents

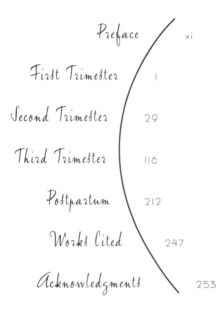

We are asked to make our most
serious and intimate commitments with
very little idea of how long they will last, or what
will be required of us. The ordinary demands of a
pregnancy, for example, require a woman to find the
strength to give birth to a child who, even if it is healthy, will
need daily nurturing for years, who will most likely devalue and
rebel against that nurture in adolescence, and who will eventually leave home for schooling, work, and a marriage of her own.
At the deepest level, a pregnant woman must find the courage to
give birth to a creature who will one day die, as she herself
must die. And there are no promises, other than the love of
God, to tell us that this human round is anything but
futile.

Kathleen Norris,

THE QUOTIDIAN MYSTERIES:
LAUNDRY, LITURGY, AND
"WOMEN'S WORK"

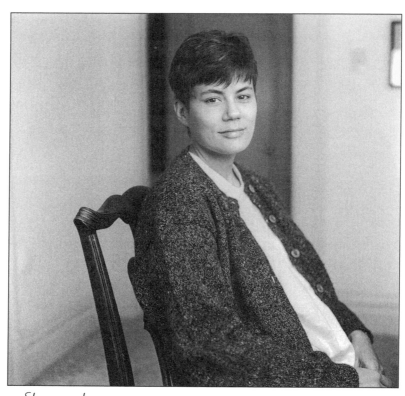

Eleven weeks pregnant.

Preface

I didn't mean to get pregnant when I did, and then, after I found out I was pregnant, I didn't plan to write a book about it. Rather, I began to write about it, to and for myself, in my journal. I'd been keeping journals since I was a girl of ten, so when I discovered I was pregnant, accidentally and to my great anxiety, I naturally turned to my notebook to record and explore this shocking turn my life had taken.

My acquaintance Charlee Brodsky and I had been looking for a joint project for a long time, one that would use my skills as a nonfiction writer and hers as a documentary photographer. Once through my initial shock, at about eight or nine weeks pregnant, I emailed Charlee with my news and apologies that we'd have to further put off working together, because I was going to have a baby. Charlee posted back with congratulations on my pregnancy, and with the suggestion that maybe it wasn't the end of our work—maybe it was the beginning.

We agreed it would be the story of a pregnant woman in her ordinary life, with Charlee shooting weekly photographs of my developing body and me continuing to record the process in my journal. When I think back on it now, after more than two years of mothering, our idea of making my pregnancy our subject reminds me of the way women writers and artists have had to seize opportunities to create within the limited spaces family life allows. Having been a mother for more than ten years, Charlee is used to looking close to home for her subject matter—so it is really not surprising that she decided to make a friend's pregnancy the subject of her work. In this case, my belly would be her dominant point of focus, but she also wanted to capture my moods, relationships, the context of my days.

For my part, I began to apply my work habits as a journalist and nonfiction writer to my long-time private habit of writing a journal. I began to research, observe, and record more closely the effects of pregnancy on my body, mind, and spirit. As my husband, Nick, and I started letting our news out, I discovered that I wasn't the only one I knew who was pregnant with a first child. My good friend Luisa was due ten days after me, and almost unbelievably my only sister, Judy, was due the day before me. It turned out that circumstance had given me other women's experiences — both very different from my own — to observe and share.

Early in my second trimester, Charlee began to bring me contact sheets from previous shoots — three, four, five dozen pictures, all of me, pregnant. I was disconcerted to see, from the outside, how much my body was growing. The image of the pregnant woman is largely absent from our visual culture of television, magazines, billboards, and websites. Over time, though, the pictures became a reassuring point of reference. *You are here — this is real,* they seemed to say, helping me make peace with the dramatic changes that pregnancy initially wreaks on a woman's sense of herself and her life in her body.

Meanwhile, in my journal I rolled with the changes, charting the swings and plateaus between deep anxiety and growing optimism about becoming a mother. I had been a wreck for the first six weeks after those two little lines turned pink on the early pregnancy test. I felt bloated, sore in my breasts, troubled in my mind, and doubtful in my heart that I could do well the enormous daily job of mothering. At the same time that I was so afraid, I was also exhilarated by this unexpected development. I had always wanted to have a child, and I felt as if a seed that had been dormant inside me had suddenly burst its casing. I could feel the seedling struggling toward daylight, full of growth and possibility. I perceived the physical rush of my fertility, but I was so scared and conflicted that I sometimes felt irreconcilably divided within myself: *I want this so much, but can I do it? I want this so much, but I'm so disgusted with the way it's making me feel.*

At the time, I criticized myself for feeling so torn. Why couldn't I just be happy, as I imagined most women are when they find out they're pregnant? Since then I've learned that many women experience mixed feelings—it's just not all that acceptable to express them. Recently, as part of my work as a publications consultant, I was interviewing a leader in the hospice movement who has worked for decades as a family physician in the rural West; when I mentioned this project and my early conflicted feelings about pregnancy, he told me, "I've helped a lot of pregnant women and delivered many babies, and I've rarely seen a pregnancy that didn't start out with a great deal of ambivalence." My midwives told me the same thing, and they encouraged me to keep writing, because most women, they said, don't feel comfortable even acknowledging—much less expressing—mixed or negative feelings about pregnancy, even to their partners.

And what about to their own mothers? I didn't feel I could admit such feelings to my mother. It wasn't just because I had a strained relationship with her, or because our ways of communicating were so different. I felt uncomfortable confiding my contradictory feelings to her because of the contradictory nature of pregnancy itself, especially for an eldest daughter pregnant for the first time. I wanted this woman whose body I'd come from—the woman I'd made into a mother—to take care of me, to give me advice and tell me everything was going to be all right. At the same time, I felt a strong desire to "do" pregnancy and motherhood in my own ways. I longed for her comfort, yet I also felt that to ask for and accept it would be tacitly to say that I was going to mother my child the same way my mother had mothered me. Some of those ways, I was beginning to see, I didn't want to reenact. So the passages in my journal about my mother explore themes of our affinity and separation. I think many first-time pregnant women go through similar exploration — often not wholly consciously, because it is implicit in our culture that it is disloyal, even shameful to want to revise with your own child your childhood experience of "mother-hood," of your mother. Yet this individuation is built into the process, and I believe it ought not to be shameful to become conscious of and to express honestly any feeling that is part of life's journey.

While texts celebrating pregnant women's happiness and anticipation abound, the experience of a pregnant woman's anxiety and deep sense of self-division is largely absent from the popular literature for pregnant women. The day I discovered I was pregnant, I went to a bookstore, skulking in the "pregnancy and childbirth" section, not wanting anyone I knew to see me shopping there. With no idea what changes might be in store, and reluctant at that time to confide in any-one but my husband, I scoured the shelves for companionship. What I wanted was a book of women's stories about pregnancy, preferably in their own voices. What I found were, essentially, "how-to" manuals dic-tating the best ways to be pregnant, full of advice from "experts." Then there were the glossy magazines with soft-focus images of apparently unpregnant models.

So it became the work of my journal, in connection with Charlee's pictures, to make sense of the contradictory and mysterious changes that were happening to me, and to Judy and Luisa, my companions in first-time pregnancy. In addition, as the weekly photo shoots piled up,

Charlee and I began to relax into friendly conversation. I learned that she had several times become pregnant but had been unable to carry these very much wanted pregnancies to term. She told me about her decision to adopt two babies, and about her approach to mothering the girls while also maintaining a university position and an independent life as an artist. She learned how I—whose life choices and circumstances are so different from my own mother's—was struggling to reimagine the role of "mother."

As the months went by, just as Charlee had shown her photographs to me, and as I was beginning to "show" in my pregnancy, I began to show this journal to others: at first to Nick and Charlee, to my pregnant friends, and to the midwives at our birth center. Eventually, long after my son was born, Charlee and I began doing readings, slide shows, and exhibits of our work.

In all the years I'd kept a journal, I'd never shared it with anyone. But this was different. Still a private space of self-examination, my journal had also become an account of pregnancy itself, as a shared process among women. I've come to see how well the journal form goes with the story of pregnancy, in its dailiness and intimacy, its succession of episodes and constant interruptions (from hunger pangs, bathroom calls, kicks from the inside), as the mother's work will be for years to come. While the photographs provide a linear narrative of the body's inexorable progress to a predictable ending, in the journal the mind and feelings blaze their own circuitous path, to an ending which is also another beginning. The Jungian analyst Jean Shinoda Bolen makes the analogy in her book on women's midlife journeys, *Crossing to Avalon:* "Pregnancy is like the creativity that comes from making a descent into one's own depth, in which the person is changed in the process of bringing forth the work—creative work that comes out of the soul and is the child of it."

Close to the end, what made it natural to share the journal, and finally to seek to publish it, is the way one's pregnancy becomes a public process. The belly stands out on the front of you, an obvious sign, not only of your sexuality, but of your simultaneous ordinariness and difference: you got pregnant. Being pregnant opens you to other people, especially to other women, and to complete strangers as well as those you know intimately. At what other moment in life do relatives and strangers alike feel entitled to stare at your body, give you little knowing smiles, pat your belly, ask you personal questions—when you're due, what sex your baby is, and whether you're going to breastfeed—and then jump in with their own blood-and-guts tales of childbirth?

People (again, especially women) seem to love stories about being pregnant and birthing children, perhaps because the work and images of it derive from our collective unconscious and our common origins. Each year, in America alone, roughly 4 million women carry pregnancies to term. The story of pregnancy and childbirth is one that binds us all, and stories serve our culture, in Terry Tempest Williams's words, as "the umbilical cord that connects the past, present, and future. . . . Story binds us to community."

Navel-Gazing is a compilation of such stories, told in words and photographs, about a process that begins in bewilderment and unfamiliarity and ends—when all goes well, as it did for Luisa, Judy, and me—in a flood of recognition and love. Along the way, *Navel-Gazing* narrates the ordinary events of pregnancy and their emotional impact: visits to physicians and midwives; telling family and friends; hearing the baby's heartbeat; feeling the baby move; seeing the baby on sonogram; dealing with the physical discomforts of pregnancy (hormone swings, sleepless nights, morning sickness, fainting spells, chronic heartburn, shortness of breath, and all the rest of it); hearing other women's stories of pregnancy and loss of pregnancy; laboring and giving birth; the newness of caring for a tiny person; regaining strength, fitness, and sexuality; envisioning the future. These stories make up a narrative that, like pregnancy itself, gains momentum and urgency as it moves toward a conclusion that is part miracle — out of one person comes two — part contradiction: pregnancy is the beginning and ending of what feels like almost everything in a woman's life.

We need to explore and articulate the conflicts and joys we experience when, as Kathleen Norris writes, we make such an "intimate commitment" with so little knowledge of what we're getting into. Our hope in sharing these common stories and images is both to demystify and to affirm the demanding and beautiful process of becoming a mother.

First Trimester

I'm pregnant.

I hardly know how to go on. Imagine — I am pregnant.

I found out yesterday. I took an eight-dollar pregnancy test, which involved sticking a plastic strip between my legs and peeing on it. The strip had two pink lines: pregnant. Just one pink line would have been a false alarm. But within the three minutes the test guaranteed, the second pink line appeared, darkening even as I prayed for it not to. I blinked and blinked, hoping for it to fade, but it didn't.

I stood at the foot of the stairs, told Nick, and had a panic attack. Hyperventilating, crying, the whole bit, and ever since, about every three to five hours, I have another one.

"I'm sorry," I kept telling him. "I'm sorry, I didn't mean it." All my adult life, I'm the one who's been taking care of the contraception.

"What do you mean?" he asked, peering into my face, his hands holding my shoulders, "this is a *good* thing."

"Oh my God," I wept, "it's a disaster."

So I called Nan in West Virginia. She was so happy — keeping it in check, because she could tell how upset I was, but she was happy. And told me to write everything down.

Feeling it's a crime to bring a new child into the world when there are so many children (and people, of whatever age) who need to be cared for, and have no one. My work on adoption with the Kellogg Foundation has taught me half a million kids in this country alone need to be adopted, and can't find permanent families.

I could have an abortion. I have the option. I don't think I can bring myself to have one, though. To me, it's a person. Not because of all the Catholic indoctrination, but because I can feel the change in my body. Not that I feel sick. I don't (perhaps this forecasts something good?). But there must be something big and important going on inside my body. My period has always come, every single month, since I was fourteen. For eighteen years. And this month, it didn't.

I wish it would.

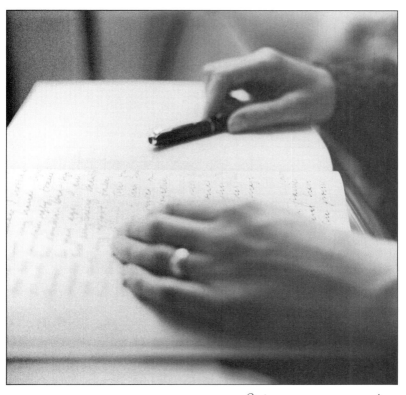

Writing in my journal.

I keep sneaking off to the bathroom to check my panties. They stay clean.

It's not that I don't want to have kids that's making me so upset. It's that I couldn't make this decision by myself. I just couldn't make it. I *wanted* to make it—I *wanted* to be able to say, to myself, to Nick, "OK—it's time, I'm ready, let's do it." But I couldn't.

Other women do it that way. Other women spend months charting their basal body temperature, trying to get pregnant, and then feel happy about it when it happens. Not me. I'm sleepless. Afraid that I will never read or write again. I read Michele Murray's diary this morning, which was probably a mistake. It *was* a mistake. She loved her kids, yeah, but she was ambivalent about motherhood, and she never made as much of her talents as she wanted to. But her time was the 1950s and '60s. I tell myself that times have changed, but it's hard to believe. I don't believe it. Even though Nick is happy and looking forward to having a baby. Even though I *know* he will share the work, I feel like I'm going to lose my whole way of life.

I called Janey this morning and cried all over her, and asked her just to promise me it wasn't the end of my life, and that I would still write. She laughed and told me my life would be *better*. That I couldn't imagine it, but it would—that I would still write—that having children was the best thing she'd ever decided to do. But Janey and Nan are both optimists. Nan said outright that being pregnant, if I can manage to give in to its demands, will be an exercise in my development as an optimist—something I've never been, never imagined I could be.

Saw Helen today. Her face when I told her I'm pregnant! It was like standing at the top of a mountain and watching a weather front move across the valley below. Happiness, confusion, pride. As my therapist she has helped me grow in so many ways these past six years. She told me she's proud of me.

We talked about everything, all the chaotic feelings and fears and bullshit. She reminded me that I've spoken about having children ever since I first came to her (I was so young then — only twenty-six). I'd forgotten.

It's a relief to have someone who truly *listens* to you. I told her stuff I'd never tell anyone else, except Nick — maybe not even him. I told her I'm afraid of not loving the kid. I told her that, since last year, when Nick started thinking about teaching in the Study Abroad program in London, I've sort of secretly imagined living in London with a baby. Now that's what's going to happen — if I carry this through. We will go to London with a baby. She encouraged me to let myself be carried away. To imagine next winter in London as a time when I can surrender myself to the baby. Not forever; just for a while.

The best thing she said was that I'm a good listener and will be able to listen to my child. She also reminded me that I know the pitfalls of making motherhood my entire work life. I have a work life. I know it's better for the kid to see me working and doing my own life, so that he or she can do its own.

I have serious doubts about my ability to be a mother. The idea keeps cropping up in the back of my mind that I could have an abortion. It's a relief to know that, if it gets too crazy and I discover that I'm just not cut out to do this, there are ways that I could get out of it. I have about two months before I hit the second trimester and that possibility expires.

✋

Saw the doctor today. Pretty ironic that, after all these years of going to a family planning center in downtown Pittsburgh to get my checkups and contraception, I just three months ago picked a new gynecologist at the university medical center who also happens to be an OB and is based at Pittsburgh's big women's hospital. They wouldn't let me see the woman I saw for my Pap test three or four months ago, because she's no longer delivering babies — she has kids of her own and doesn't want to be on call that unpredictably. But there are two others in the group — a man and a woman.

The receptionist hadn't wanted me to come in. "Jeez, you're not even two months pregnant," she told me, and she tried to give me an appointment for next month. But I've had a migraine since yesterday, and I needed to know what kind of medication I can take for the pain. "How about *today?*" I insisted. "Or tomorrow?"

The doctor examined me and said my cervix was soft and my uterus enlarged — about five weeks pregnant. He set the due date at September 24.

He spent about fifteen minutes with me. I asked all the questions I could think of, and he answered them in a kind of monotone without meeting my eyes. I just lay on the table in a stupor, with the ice pack one of the nurses had given me pressed against my right temple.

He gave me a prescription for Tylenol with codeine. I've never taken codeine and have no idea how it will work. Won't it hurt the baby? He said codeine has been around for decades and decades and that I shouldn't be afraid to take it.

✼

We told Mom and Dad last night. It was Dad's birthday, and we went out to their house in the suburbs for dinner. I thought our news would be a nice birthday present, and I felt pretty calm about the idea of telling them, but as we all looked at each other over empty dessert plates I found myself starting to tremble. "We have some news for you," I ventured, and I told them that in September we expect to be having a child. Mom's jaw dropped and they said nothing for a full minute. Then they burst into smiles and congratulations.

Sitting at their kitchen table, I thought how different this discussion was from our big argument of ten years ago, at that very same table, though last night I was—literally and figuratively—sitting on the other side. Ten years ago: the beginning of my too-long-delayed separation from my mother, the beginning (I can see now) of her realization that I was not going to do life the same way she had done life. I was not going to marry the first man I had fallen in love with; I was not going to marry a Catholic. I was not going to eschew contraception; I was not going to sleep in my own apartment till my wedding night; I was not going to stay in the church. I was not going to go to all lengths to avoid making mistakes; I was, in fact, going to make some big mistakes. I was not anymore going to set an "example" for my younger sister, Judy. I wasn't going to be a "good" girl; I wasn't even going to spin my story that way. I remember driving back to West Virginia and sitting in the newsroom one night before my 11 P.M. deadline, in tears, and telling Nan about the argument. She was my editor, but we'd also become close friends in the six or seven months we'd worked together. I had to talk to *someone;* she's eleven years older than I, just old enough to have participated in the remnants of the late-sixties counterculture; she had made choices that differed in the extreme from her mother's. She told me then that it sounded like the wound was so deep that a grandchild would be the only way to heal it.

"Did I *say* that?" she said the other day on the phone. "God, how arrogant of me."

But she might have been right. I suspected it myself, even before she said it. I was only twenty-two then, but I knew it might take me bringing another life into the world—another person that was part of their own flesh and blood; taking a lifelong job with the unmistakable whiff of tradition and convention about it—for us to get close to each other again.

🖑

Called Luisa, another former colleague, the other day and told her I'm pregnant. "Well, guess what," she whispered. "I am, too."

I had an inkling she might be! She said last fall that she and E.J. were going to begin trying in November. She's due October 4.

I'm so glad to have a friend to go with me through this process. It sounds like I'm having less trouble so far than she is. She's got some morning sickness. And she's been spotting blood, which is freaking her out, though they did an ultrasound and everything looks OK.

My clothes are already too tight. I'm not eating more than usual, though last week I had an irresistible cheese craving and ate mostly cheese—cheddar cheese on crackers; slices of Monterey Jack with peppers; that "cheese-and-salsa" concoction on corn chips. Cheese is the only craving I've had so far (except for the craving for jalapeño peppers along with the cheese—I found myself popping them right out of the jar and into my mouth—maybe whoever it is in there is coming from a past life in Mexico).

My breasts are growing out of my bras.

I'm writing this in the ladies' lounge of the Park Terrace Hotel near Dupont Circle, in D.C., where we've been for the past three days. My jeans are so tight I can barely breathe. The only way I can move with any comfort is if I skip a meal, but then I feel weak and nauseated. When I eat, I feel fat. The books say pregnancy is not the time to try to *lose* weight.

Do I really need a *book* to tell me that?

So relieved—I got a digital scale, and it says I've only gained one or two pounds. I keep thinking that I'm only in the first month, when I'm probably six or seven weeks pregnant—nearly two months. So I'm supposed to be putting on a pound a month until four months or so.

Today I told Jeri. I felt so nervous about telling her. I've been working for her as a subcontract writer for the past two years, and have known her for eight. She's one of my best friends, and her mentorship has been so important to me; our high level of trust as friends and fellow writers makes working together a very smooth and enjoyable

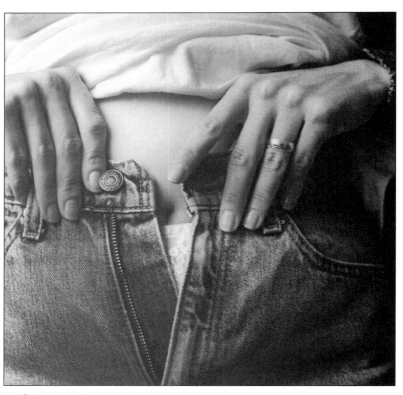

Eleven weeks pregnant.

process. But because we work with such high-level foundation people and our contracts have increasingly large bottom lines, it felt like a significant step to let her know I'm pregnant. I waited until today because I had a big deadline for her, and I wanted to prove that pregnancy wasn't going to prevent me from doing our work and doing it well. Jeri wasn't surprised at all by the news. "You've been talking about this for a long time," she said. That's what Helen said. I guess I hadn't admitted to myself that I'd been giving it such serious thought.

Jeri said she was glad for us. "You know, it may not be politically correct to say this," she said, "but compared to all this" — she gestured at our work, spread out on the table — "raising a kid is the greatest work you can ever do. I really believe it."

Both kinds of work are good, though, and I want to do them both, even though I have no model in my family that says it's OK to be a mother and keep up my own work. I remember Mom saying that women who put their kids in child care so they could work either were being selfish or were unwilling to accept a lower standard of living, or both. "You can't have *everything*" was one of her maxims, and "Who ever said life is fair? It isn't fair." Does it have to be a choice, though? I'm not sure. I'm just trying to stick with my sense that God wouldn't give me a kid in *exchange* for all the other good work God has also given me.

❧

Von was overjoyed when I told her this afternoon that I'm pregnant. We've been having these quiet meditation groups at our house, in front of our fireplace. Sometimes there are three or four of us from our Quaker Meeting, sitting in silence for an hour or so, but today it was just me and Von. Afterward, when I told her I had been contemplating the child I was expecting to have in eight months, her face looked like it might explode, like fireworks. I asked her not to tell anyone else in Meeting but said she could tell Dale, and they took us out to dinner, their treat. Dale even ordered a bottle of champagne. It was a real celebration.

I felt awkward accepting anything alcoholic, even though no one can tell I'm pregnant. I felt like I might be carded all over again — a big, scarlet "PG" on my driver's license.

"There's nothing wrong with a small glass of champagne," Von said, and pushed a flute in front of me. "When I was having Carter, my doctor told me a glass of port in the evening would relax me and relax the uterus. Of course, that was twenty-four years ago, but *some* things don't change."

☙

I cannot *believe* this, but Judy's also pregnant. What's more, she's due September 23 — the day before me. What are the odds that sisters would be due within a day of each other? She made me promise not to tell anyone else in the family, though she told Mom and Dad a couple of days before we told them. Tim doesn't want anyone but parents — grandparents, that is! — to know until Judy hits the three-month mark. He's hardly even acknowledging it himself. I guess that, as an OB, he's seen just about every problem in the book.

No wonder Mom and Dad were so shell-shocked — no wonder Mom couldn't say anything — their two first grandkids coming at the same time — maybe even on the same day!

I had called Judy tonight to tell her the news, and to get Tim's advice on the codeine. When I told her I'm pregnant, Judy just laughed and laughed.

"Why are you laughing?" I said.

"Because I am, too," she said. I thought she was joking. Then I remembered that she and Tim had been trying for several months.

Charlee is going to shoot pictures of me once a week, beginning in the middle of March when Nick and I get back from our spring break in Arizona.

❧

Phoenix, Arizona.

Nick and I went to the Native American festival downtown. Booths with loads of jewelry and kachina dolls, painted pottery and rugs and hides made into pouches, moccasins, belts, hangings. The sun was high and hot, and I was beginning to feel like I had a lead ball in my belly. I was going to suggest we escape into the cool air of the Heard Museum when he said, "Can I show you this piece I love?" He led me to a place in the festival where, on a makeshift plywood table, sat "Clown Seeing the World Through New Eyes." A black-and-terracotta-striped clay man—a joker with corn-shuck tongues of "fire" blooming from the top of his head, peering at the world through "glasses" made from thumbs and forefingers.

But the piece I liked was a bronze of a woman sitting naked, leaning on her right hand with her left hand tucked between her thighs and her head bent over her right shoulder. One lock of hair fell over her

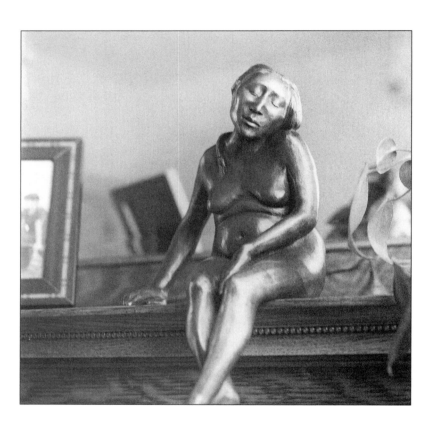

right collarbone. Her brown legs were crossed at the ankles, the toes spread slightly. Her breasts pointed downward and spread to either side of her round belly. She was so relaxed that a crease formed in her belly underneath her breasts.

"What's the name of this one?" I asked the sculptor. All the other statues had title cards. As soon as I said it I could feel my eyes stinging, as though I might cry. Maybe it's hormones, but the artist's eyes were so large and such a soft brown. She seemed to be looking below the first few layers of my skin, making me feel as though she recognized me from somewhere.

"A Moment in Time," she answered. She looked about my age. She kept her eyes on my face, and I did cry a little bit after all.

"I'm sorry," I told her, "it's just that the statue is so beautiful. And also, I'm pregnant."

She continued to look up at my face from where she sat, on a rock in the parking lot, her arms clasped around her knees. "I see now," she said. "When I first saw you, I said to myself, 'I wonder who that woman is?' There seems to me a warm glow around your body."

Oh, right. The pregnant woman's "glow." But her brown eyes seemed so sincere. "Maybe the glow came when I was looking at her," I said, pointing to the statue.

"Maybe it's inside you," she said gently.

I sat on the asphalt of the parking lot with her and we talked for a while. Her name is Roxanne Swentzell, and her studio is at Santa Clara Pueblo in New Mexico. Her sculptures have gone all over the world; one of them was part of a Heard Museum exhibit that went to the

British Museum. Yet for all the public attention she receives, it's "the deep, hidden life," as Michele Murray writes, that continues to fascinate her and inspire her work. She calls herself "a sculptor of the human emotions." "I want to show people a different part of themselves than they usually show," she says. "I keep believing that if I keep reaching those depths in myself, it's going to help others reach that, too."

She told me some things about the Pueblo Indian concept of "mother." " 'Mother' is anyone who takes care of people and who protects the earth. So even a man can be 'mother.' It's a term of respect and honor, not denigration," she said.

We just bought the bronze statue. "I'm so happy the baby will see her and grow up with her in our house," I told Roxanne. When I said this, she put her arms around me. Nick suggested we name the statue "Clara" after the pueblo where she was made. The statue means "mother" to me and makes me feel less afraid of being pregnant, bearing a baby, and raising a child.

Sedona, Arizona.

At four thousand feet the sun is warm and sharp.

We hiked on the red rock mountains. There were all these signs in town advertising Sedona's "energy vortexes"—we even picked up maps pinpointing the locations of the vortexes and brochures asking us to join the many "vortex tours" on offer, but we just went off by ourselves. We drove up a canyon, pulled off at a trailhead, and began climbing a mountain. Halfway up we paused to catch our breath (even though I've gained just four pounds or so, it feels much harder to breathe). We sat for a while, holding hands, mesmerized by the beauty and strength of the red mountain opposite ours that rose sheer from the valley floor below.

We made love a few paces off the trail, behind a boulder and some brush. Then we went back to our spot and watched the mountain some more before hiking back down to the car.

Hmm, maybe we stumbled onto a vortex? — I don't think so, though it was pretty passionate. The sun seems stronger here than at home — when you take off your shirt (which was delicious, up on that mountain), the sun penetrates your skin and fires you up somehow. There was definitely something about the huge red rocks, the white clouds scudding low overhead, and the dry, pure air that opened our senses.

On the walk I was thinking that, if I'm going to have this kid, I need to come up with my own idea of how to be a mother that's based on something other than the anxiety that seemed to color Mom's life, and that I learned from her. The fear that seemed always present under her surfaces that we'd turn out all wrong, and she'd be a failure.

I'm realizing lately that when I think of "mother," I think of Mom, but I also think of Grandma, Daddy's mother, who took care of anybody who showed up on her doorstep. One of her chief pleasures was making delicious food for her family, which extended well beyond the walls of her house. She had a hot temper, but she always let her anger go. She was always poor, but she never worried about money. She lost two husbands and two children and her house in the Great Depression, but she always trusted that the world would take care of her if she took care of her little bit of the world.

My image of Mom galvanizes me, "For God's sake, do the very best you can." My image of Grandma soothes me. "Don't worry about the baby, honey, it'll be all right," I hear her say. "Just love it and be happy, and God will help you one day at a time."

Being "even-tempered," the Heard exhibit said, is one of the most valued qualities in a good woman among Indian societies. The Croatian word for "good woman" is *kuma*, which where Dad came from was usually taken to mean "godmother." Dad's side of the family is Croatian — Grandma came over on a boat in 1909. Everybody called Grandma Kuma Jennie, whether she'd held them at the baptismal font or not.

I'm certain I will yell at my kid's disobedience, at the constant mess family life makes of the house and the schedule, at my entrapment within the house. I'd like to be as certain that I can achieve victories as small and simple as keeping an even temper — most of the time — making good food, letting go of my anxiety. Trusting God to take care of me so I can take care of my family. Daring to be happy.

Flagstaff, Arizona.

Hiked for a few hours in the Grand Canyon yesterday. We hadn't really planned to hike and didn't even bring boots, but once we were there the opportunity seemed too good. The south rim was icy and slick in spots and I had no hiking boots, so for the first time ever on a trail I felt nervous and insecure. It would have been easy to fall and break a bone or even slip over the edge in some spots. I felt energetic, though, despite my growing belly. No matter how I eat and how much I exercise, my belly continues to grow. I'm not used to being out of control of this body of mine. I'm only ten weeks pregnant—just a fourth of the way there—yet I can fit into none of my jeans except the big old black ones that I never used to wear. Sometimes I panic at having the body in which I've grown so comfortable stolen away from me, even temporarily. The problem is I don't believe it's going to be temporary.

I think once the weather warms up at home and I can get out into the new garden I want to build, I'll be less obsessed with my body. Working with dirt always calms and cheers me. Even now, despite anxiety, I feel healthy and happy, and ready to get back to life at home.

※

Jerome, Arizona.

Finished Kingsolver's collection of essays last night. This holiday I came away with only one book, instead of my usual half dozen, so I actually finished the one I brought. She writes that she can't even remember how she used to write before her daughter made "a grown-up" out of her. I identified with this statement. In the six or seven weeks that I've had this other person to think about and care for, it has become even more important to me that I have work of my own. I also have a sense of urgency about doing my work whenever I get the chance. Before I got pregnant, I felt I had all the time in the world to do a given piece of work. If I didn't "feel" like working, I didn't bother to push myself too hard. Now I have a sense of an impending deadline that will change my whole life once it arrives.

I bought the baby a Navajo dream-catcher yesterday. I chose it carefully — buttery deerskin with pink and white beads and three feathers. The first item in what I'm sure will be a large accumulation of stuff. We're going to hang it over the crib — when we get around to buying a crib.

I've been having strange dreams — not exactly nightmares, but just full of strangeness. Last night's was full of canyon imagery: red rocks, arroyos of yellow and red-brown and red-black, and sheer cliffs of yellow sandstone and gray limestone. I was climbing, and suddenly the earth shifted and I fell, tumbling through an opening in the earth. No pain, but the terror of a sheer drop, and a sense of failure. At not having read the signs correctly. At being stuck in a land so unfamiliar and inhospitable to the hiker, the curious wanderer.

We heard the baby's heartbeat yesterday. It was our three-month checkup and we had the woman OB partner again, who doesn't like to hang around and spend a lot of time — neither does the guy — but she put on her gloves and measured me from inside and out and said my uterus was about as big as a grapefruit, "twelve- to thirteen-week size."

"How big is it when it's not pregnant?" I asked.

"The size of a pear," she said. "We go by fruit here." Then in silence she slicked my belly with gel. While I was thinking about the size of my uterus, and how much stuff it must be pushing out of the way, she pointed to a spot three inches below my navel, the spot our T'ai Ch'i teacher used to call "the center of all energy in the body," and said quietly, "It's right about here." She stuck the end of a plastic tube against

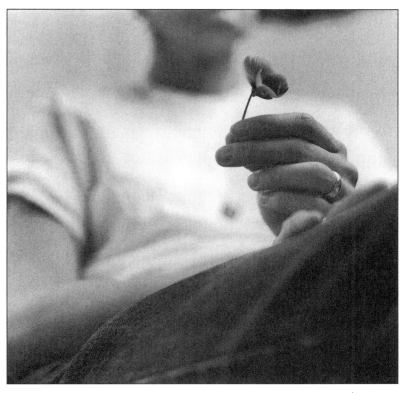

Pandy.

that spot and through the fuzzy speaker came a muffled thud—*poof, poof, poofpoofpoofpoof.*

"There it is," she said.

"That's it?" I said, my neck straining and static pouring through the speaker. Just as I can't do *anything* alone anymore, I couldn't sit up or speak without the Doppler picking up my noise. I lay back again and, as Nick stared, the static fell back into a steady beat, as though being transmitted from outer space to be picked up by a receiver in my belly. It sounded out quietly but insistently in the white room.

"About 163 beats per minute," she said. "When they're this small, we expect them to be fast. It's working away." As it will for the next seventy-five years, on average—till 2073.

PoofpoofpoofpoofTHHHHHH—"Oh, it just moved," she said, smiling like a diviner, rod in hand, standing over found water.

"It *moved?*" we said.

"It's bouncing around in there," she said.

❧

Back home.

I think it's a girl. Dreamed last night I was carrying her. "My baby." What will she be like? If it's a girl, what if we just reenact everything I know about mother-daughter relationships? Makes me think of that line in Margaret Drabble's *The Millstone:* "Gradually I began to realize . . . that unless I took great pains to alienate her she would go on liking me, for a couple of years at least." Maybe I could manage that, if it's a girl. If it's a boy, we'll automatically get along great. No competition.

This pregnancy is changing me already. I wake and don't dread the day. Imagine going through most of one's life dreading each day, all the possible fuckups that could happen, and then all of a sudden not dreading anything anymore. That's the way I feel. Not because I feel like the kid has given me "a purpose" in life. (Though, I admit it, I now have a large project that needs attention and work, and that's what I'm good at—seeing a project through to completion.) It's also everything I'm learning. About how the body works. About being out of control of other people.

And get this—the person who's teaching me this is living inside my body.

"I had the worst day today," Judy told me on the phone last night.

"Why?" I asked.

"I spent the *whole day* writing," she said. My dream. "And I'd rather, like, iron a *hundred* of Tim's shirts than write."

Nick is in Yorkshire. The family called from Leeds at 7:30 this morning to offer congratulations about the baby. The Baby, The Baby, is that all anybody will care about from now on? I don't understand this whole phenomenon. Why are people who reproduce to be automatically congratulated? Why is it assumed to be a "miracle," a "blessing," a "bundle of joy"?

In our case it was a mistake. An accident. We were at the end of a two-day argument on Christmas holiday and groped for each other in the shower, tired of fighting, desperate for some peace, for even momentary connection. When I stepped (weak-kneed) out of the tub, dripping, I thought, "I'm sure I've done it this time." And I had. I'd done it. Done myself in. If I remember correctly, it was only *afterward* that Nick said, "Did you have your diaphragm in?" "It's only five days since my period started," I said carelessly. "We're safe." But we were not safe. Now I have to pay the price for the rest of my life. Forever, until I die or the kid dies before me, I have to worry about and care for this other person that I did not even ask for.

Moreover, this person will not even be guaranteed to love me. I have to do all this because I reproduced myself, and because the cultural belief—and it is just a belief, isn't it?—is that babies are "bundles of joy."

Hearing the heartbeat, and the surprise and wonder I felt at that moment (and for the rest of the evening), seems to me now a narcissistic daydream. A naive buy-in to the prevailing cultural belief.

I could still have an abortion. That's still an option. But look at all the people we've told. How would we explain it? We'd have to tell the truth and hurt everyone we've already told. Or, we'd have to lie and say I lost the baby. And not only would I have to live through the abortion, I'd have to live with having caused yet more hurt in my family, or with the lie.

Then I think: What if I'm not cut out to be a mother? What if I'm too selfish, too into my work to give so much time to another person? And how am I supposed to know whether I'm capable before I even try? What's worse, living through the abortion and the explanation to everyone we've told—or ruining the life of another whole person because you're not able to be a good mother?

It doesn't matter how many people know we're pregnant or how we'd explain an abortion. That's not the point. The point is, I've become invested in this person. Nick has become invested in this person. Can I say I love this person? I don't know. I can only say that this person, as tiny and unformed as it is, is already big and powerful enough to have changed our lives together. Which means I have to admit: however ambivalent I feel about being pregnant and however just plain scared I feel about being a mother, on some level I must want to do this work. On some level, I must want to try. That must mean that I'll find the wherewithal bit by bit. I'll make it up as I go along, however impossible that seems now. I'll fake it till I make it. I'm already doing it.

I've figured out why I'm so torn about being pregnant. I flashed on the reason yesterday just as I was running out the door to a meeting, and I had no time to write it down.

The discovery is: I don't believe anything I do will change anyone's life or attitude. I am a pessimist. Not only that—I *choose* to be one. It's not just the way life is; I choose to see it this way.

I began to come to this conclusion two days ago when Nan, my friend from West Virginia, came to visit. She and I sat in the kitchen talking politics—welfare, education, health care. I was saying things are just as bad now as they ever have been, or worse; and she was saying things are better. She said people are eating, there's food enough to go around—which I disputed—and that we'll always have the poor. "The poor you will always have with you," she said, quoting that place in the Bible. Nan *never* quotes the Bible. This made me take her really seriously.

As I began to stick with the position I was taking—"We're as bad off now as we've ever been, or worse"—I started to experience, in a kind of clinical way, what it has meant for me all these years to choose a pessimistic viewpoint. I'd always thought pessimism was sort of mandatory—the Roman Catholic "suffer now for paradise later" mentality I grew up with kind of left me convinced I couldn't change anything on earth. I've always doubted I could change anyone's mind, influence anyone's perspective, or make anyone's life better. In fact, I've always suspected, despite a pile of evidence to the contrary, that I've made Nick's life worse, more of a care and a trouble than it would have been were he on his own or with a woman who is older and more mature than I. These things have always seemed to me to be the facts of life—unarticulated but nonetheless binding.

Yesterday, though, I realized that these things are not facts. They are ideas that I choose to adopt. I realized what probably everybody else on earth already knows—that people choose to be pessimists. All these years, I've been *choosing* to be a pessimist. On the heels of that, of course, I asked myself—like I always do these days, practically down to every bite of food I eat—what this means for the baby.

What does my being a pessimist mean for the baby? Living the life of a pessimist means I don't believe that, if I take care of my kid out of love, he or she is going to love me back. Money-back guarantee. This is

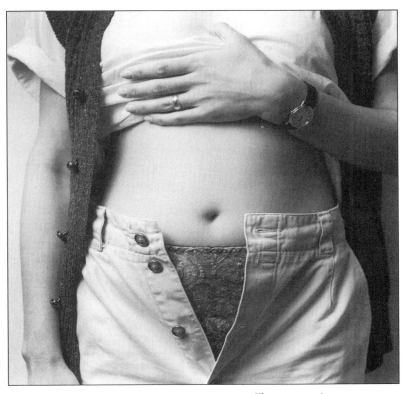

Thirteen weeks pregnant.

one of the most central equations about life. It's the one that most religions of the world are based on! It's karma, for God's sake! Cause and effect. What goes around, comes around. I allow it to apply to everybody in the world — except me.

The bottom line is, I'm not really sure there's a kid inside me at all — let alone that he or she is virtually guaranteed to love me.

God has a funny way of answering prayers. They always say, "Be careful what you ask for — you just might get it." Some unconscious part of my mind might have said a few silent prayers for me to have a kid. But if I ever — even unconsciously — got down on my knees and asked for this much psychic upheaval, I sure as hell don't remember.

Second Trimester

Today's the third shoot with Charlee and I am nervous, as usual. How should I hold my body? It's hard to relax in front of the camera. I feel like I'm under a magnifying glass. I'm not used to being someone else's subject — usually I'm the one doing the interviewing, the examining. She doesn't show any compulsion to talk, though; it's just her holding that big, square Rollei camera in front of her own belly, peering into the viewfinder, snapping the shutter button, clicking the film through its rollers. Focus . . . snap . . . click . . . focus . . . Sometimes five or ten minutes will go by without either of us saying anything, just that focus, snap, click, and her changing the film from time to time. The roll holds twelve shots, and she shoots from three to five rolls each time she comes.

When she opens the camera to change film, sometimes I'll ask her about her girls. I knew they were adopted, but it turns out that Charlee had gotten pregnant several times but lost all the pregnancies. One was in the third month. I can now imagine how painful that must have been — and she was much clearer than I am about wanting to be a mother.

Charlee is crazy about Gillian and Ally. She loves talking about her mothering and seems to retain no regret that her kids did not come from her own body. Talk about an optimist. She seems to keep her focus on what she has.

Nan said last weekend that my pessimism will turn into optimism when I feel the baby moving. (I hate calling it "the baby." It never seems to come out of my mouth easily and I end up calling it "the kid," which makes people laugh. But I can't get my mouth around "the baby" and will be relieved when we know what sex it is and I can begin to use a gendered pronoun. I like best the phrase that Von uses — "our baby." Makes me feel like I'll have more help than just Nick's in raising it after it comes. But then Von is a child psychologist and runs a preschool that was started by Dr. Spock. She knows that, at best, it takes more than two people to raise a good kid.) Nan said I *have* to write about when it moves and tell her how it makes me feel. This won't happen till the fourth or fifth month, they say, but it is all beginning to go faster and faster and some moments it seems September will be here in no time at all. I'm not freaking out, though. I feel calm and happy.

Nick keeps saying, "You're doing so well." Others keep saying that too. As though I'm in training, or rehearsing for a big performance. Which is how the pregnancy manuals talk about it—in terms of training for a performance.

I feel strange when people tell me how well I'm doing. My lips form the appropriate thanks, but beyond that I am never sure how to respond, because I'm just doing my life—which now happens to include having a baby. At the same time, having people so frequently encourage me in that commonplace project—doing my life—feels luxurious, and I long to hear it again: "You're doing so *well.*"

Almost passed out at the session with Charlee this morning. She wanted a closeup of my neck and stood me right next to her light. I began to see stars and had no idea why I felt faint, but I had to sit down. Put my head between my knees and felt a little embarrassed, like I was not doing my job right.

So I got up too soon. We went back to it, and right away the stars came back. I tried to push on through, but a minute or two later I was on my knees and everything was black. I knew it was going to happen; at the same time, I didn't believe it. (Just like I know I'm pregnant, but I don't believe there's anybody in there.) Still, I don't see myself as the fainting-lady type. I'm not athletic, but I'm strong and fit, and what I most felt, when the stars wiped out my vision and I could no longer stand, was irritation. *What the fuck's going on here?*—a slavedriver's voice.

"I'm sorry," I told Charlee.

She wasn't bothered. For her, it was all part of the story. She snapped pictures of me lying down.

"You're just a more physical rather than rational being right now. You're a *creature,*" she said in her gentle voice. A creature. *La criatura:* Estés's Wild Woman. "As in all art," Estés writes, "she resides in the guts, not in the head."

Took a long bike ride yesterday. I felt fluid, relaxed, and lithe except for my thick midsection. (Even my breasts are getting in the way of my arms now. I'll need to buy bigger bras soon.) When I reached the garden center, just as I unhooked my helmet and shook out my hair, I ran into one of the men who works there, a guy who has always struck me as so attractive in a purely physical way. He greeted me with appreciation and I found myself wondering if he would look at me with such interest — with any interest at all — in another month or two, when my belly has become larger and round.

Are there men who recognize the sensuality in pregnancy? — not just your own husband, whose investment is obvious and emotional, but men who aren't numb to the energy for which a pregnant woman is a channel, and who see themselves as a channel for it as well, in a different way? I don't mean the jerks who feel it's their duty and calling to impregnate women. I mean men who know that we all come from the same place — between a woman's legs, between the rocking endpoints of her pelvis — and grow from there to carry that generative energy into the world.

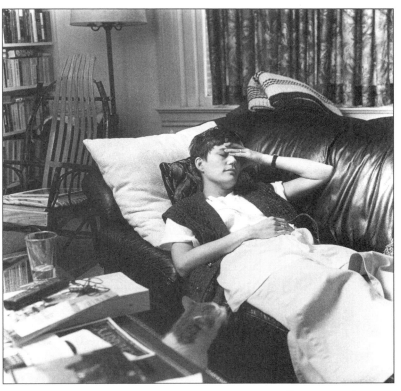

Almost passed out.

✺

Dressing for a bike ride with Von this morning, I put on an old white stretch-lace underwire bra. Nick lay in bed staring at me. These days, he can't help but stare at me as I dress.

"Nice new bra," he said.

"It's an old bra."

"Oh—nice old bra," he replied, cocking a smile: "I guess it's the breasts that are new."

✺

On the bike ride with Von, I felt a strange power in being able to ride as I always have, yet also hold another person inside me. I've been trying to imagine it—a whole being claiming residence in my body. I imagine a little person building its house, walking around. Von's unequivocal support and enthusiasm are infectious. She's ga-ga over "our baby."

We stopped at the Presbyterian church to walk their labyrinth—a mazelike path that twists and turns back on itself till it reaches a center resting place, like the eye in a hurricane. It's used for meditation and prayer. The one we walked is painted on a huge square piece of canvas. They had spread it out in the church basement, a big, gothic room that was dusky even at lunchtime, but candles glowed around the labyrinth's perimeter. It looks just like the one at Chartres Cathedral. Who would have guessed we have one right in our own back yard? I didn't even know about it till Von told me. The concept is apparently more than four thousand years old and shows up in almost every religious tradition. In medieval Europe it was supposed to represent the one true path to God, while for some Native American tribes it represented Mother Earth and was analogous to the kiva, the sacred prayer hole dug deep into the earth, the very center of which translates into *belly button navel.* There were all sorts there—students, old people, office workers who set down their briefcases and took off their shoes to walk and think or pray during their lunch hour. A much wiser choice than McDonald's, or lunch at your desk. The room was still except for the hushed shuffling of stocking feet pacing the ancient sacred path that twined toward the flower in the center, the resting place.

"We are not human beings on a spiritual path, but spiritual beings on a human path," an expert on the labyrinth writes. I thought that was good. It makes me think of this pregnancy. Nothing about my experience of it so far has been straightforward. I've had to patiently walk a path of ambivalence and uncertainty and have faith that I'll eventually make it to the center, where I can rest (at least for a moment).

It also makes me think of the kid. Where is the kid on its human path? What a stunning thing, to think that I've got a whole separate spiritual being inside me, just starting out on its long and winding (human) road.

After the walk, Von and I sat for a while in silence in the church's little brick-paved courtyard, where the dogwood and fruit trees are just beginning to bud. I noticed that I've been calmer and happier than ever. When I sit, I no longer cross my legs and swing my foot nervously. I seem to be able to relax inside my skin.

I guess any of this contentment can be attributed to the stabilized hormones of the second trimester. I was reading about hormones the other day, and it's amazing how much higher the hormone levels rise during pregnancy. Estrogen alone rises to about a thousand times its nonpregnant level. Estrogen makes the uterus grow, and progesterone develops the milk glands; progesterone is kicking in for me right now, in the second trimester. Maybe that's why I feel so happy. Progesterone is the happy hormone. It goes straight to all the body's smooth muscles — the "automatic" ones, the ones that control the life-giving functions: intestines and heart and diaphragm — and makes them relax. Instant deep relaxation — the yogi hormone.

Maybe it's hormones, and maybe it's increased exercise, and maybe it's avoiding my habitual chocolate binges, or any amount of refined sugar, or reducing caffeine. We even cut our morning tea with decaf. The changes are not just physical, though. Along with the changes in my body comes a sense of being irrevocably changed in my psyche and in my character. The body altered *forever:* breasts perhaps not forever larger, but certainly softer and more sensitive; blood vessels opened in pelvis and labia — forever opened; the sense that I myself, my body and whole being, will from now until I die be opened, less private.

This sense comes to me at moments of half-awareness — say, just before I fall asleep. It washed over me like a tide while making love with Nick the other night. We had just come from dinner. I had a belly full of baby and rich food, and I knew I wanted to be close to his body, but I wasn't sure I could respond. At first I didn't respond, though lying next to him felt so relaxing. Taking my clothes off, I felt slightly more receptive, though also embarrassed, as in the old days when I was afraid of what he would think of my body. But he always loves my body. His caresses over my broadening haunches and belly relaxed me, and I melted in his arms, grateful to be held against him. His hand moved between my thighs and suddenly I felt as though we weren't alone. I sensed the being inside me that he and I had created — out of nothing, it seems: it took me more energy and forethought two weeks ago to sow a row of peas in the garden — and I felt as though I were the place that had been prepared and sowed.

As I lay like a rumpled mountain range against his body, I felt the plates of my old self grind against each other and open, and new ground be created. I felt heaved open. Like a fault line that has withstood pressure and tension for years, and suddenly gives. It felt like a yielding to permanent change: you can't put back ground swallowed up during a fault-line movement.

Then the old metaphors of possession rose in my mind. As he kissed my breast I thought, "He's inside my body — my body's his now —" That old rhetoric of surrender and conquest. Those cultural metaphors get so deeply ingrained that they sneak up on you when you're at your least rational. This had less to do with Nick "giving it to me" than with my own willingness lately to accept the conditions of my life. I have to eat more food; my body not only is getting bigger, it *looks* bigger; I have more energy; I have — perhaps not an abundance of friends — but an abundance of affection for and from those I have; and lots of love between Nick and me. All this love just washed over me when my body responded to his. It was a giving in, a yielding to decades of absentee ownership of the place where I live: my body.

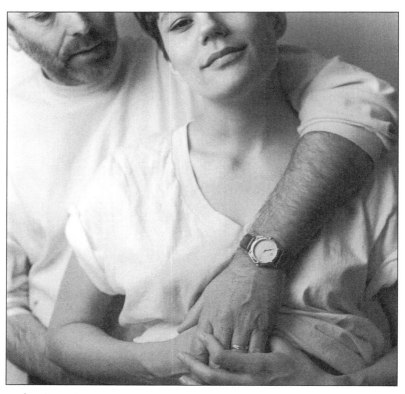

Nick and me.

So depressed yesterday that I was transported back to my pre-pregnancy self. I felt that maybe it was naive to like getting up in the morning, sentimental to be touched by the low song of the mourning dove and the sight of blue sky at our bedroom window. I couldn't make myself do anything the whole day except write a few questions for an interview, call a client, and buy groceries.

What pissed me off the most today—looking at how happy I was in the previous entry—was the suspicion that maybe, just maybe, I don't deserve to be so happy. Daydreaming about the kid has become an unconscious habit that not only makes me happy in a direct way (I enjoy it when I do it) but also accrues a lot of indirect benefits. With the kid always in the back of my mind (and on the front of my body), making me think of the future, I try harder at clearing out that dark, dusty space inside my mind—I work harder, I try harder in my relationships. I'm beginning to see a new view of the world through the windows I'm cleaning, and I have more hope.

Nan was right. I'm becoming an optimist. In just a few weeks, I've become used to feeling hopeful, and behaving in hopeful ways. Which to me right now primarily denotes the belief I can make an impact on my world; maybe not the whole world, but my world. I have already. For example, I'm helping Jeri to produce publications that change public policy. This work not only benefits the publications' "stakeholders" and makes money for me and my family, but it also supports a nurturing work situation for my colleagues—three other women I care about.

I knew all along I was doing this work, but I haven't looked at the big picture in such a positive way before.

❦

Going for a walk with Luisa tonight. She's still having problems with spotting, and she cries every day. She says she expects it to be a difficult summer. We both have gained seven pounds but, she's quick to note, she's shorter. Says her mother-in-law told her that she's going to have a girl because she's "carrying all over."

"That's a bunch of bullshit," I said.

"I don't know," she said dubiously. She's superstitious. Both of us are.

Nick and I visited my grandmother today, the day before Easter, and told her the news. She still didn't know we're having a baby. I was surprised Mom hadn't mentioned it; she's telling all her friends. "It's not *my* place to tell her," she said to me. Judy told her about her own pregnancy over the phone several weeks ago.

When we arrived, she was ensconced on her sofa. She talked for a long time about her dissatisfaction with the food at her retirement community, and various health concerns. Trying to get a word in, I said peremptorily, *"I've* got something," as though I had an illness. It was cheeky of me. Her face grew wary and Nick said, with a nervous chuckle, "No, you haven't."

"Yes I do," I retorted.

"What have you got?" she said, eyeing me narrowly.

"I've got a baby," I said coyly, thinking she'd break into a smile, maybe get up off the couch to hug us. I still need to learn that expectations are a waste of energy.

"You've *got* a baby, or you're *going to have* a baby?" she demanded.

Jeez. "I'm gonna have a baby," I corrected, and as she leaned back on the couch, her face settled into its customary complacent lines.

"When's *yours* due?" she said.

She didn't wait for me to answer before she started retelling the stories of her own two labors, the first, with Mom, lasting three days and leaving her in the hospital for another fifteen. I hadn't heard this story for ages, and in the state I'm in, it was like hearing it for the first time. I listened incredulously as she told me that the nurses refused to let her even *see* Mom for the first four days of her life. Maybe this was standard treatment then, but still: I pictured Mom as a little baby, lying all by herself in a hospital bassinet, crying after such a physical ordeal, desperate for her mother's comfort. As my grandmother swept by us on the momentum of telling her story, never asking us how we felt about our news, never glancing at Nick (whose eyes, admittedly, were sliding to a close as he reclined in her blue leather Barcalounger), I found myself thinking that the anxiety and depression of unfulfilled needs started for Mom on Day One. She was denied the birthright every baby possesses: her right, her need, to be held, stroked, gazed at, and told as soon as she came into this world how wonderful she was just for being *herself.*

It's hard to write about Mom. I thought this was just my own personal problem until I dug out Adrienne Rich when I was about six weeks pregnant. Other women sit around and read *What to Expect When You're Expecting* (which Nick and I have nicknamed *What to Expect*

When You're Expecting the Worst, because of how paranoid it makes me), but not me: I pick feminist theory. Count on Rich to say the feelings no one else wants to say, that no one else even wants to look at. The Rich book had sat unopened on my bookshelf for at least half a dozen years till one day a couple of months ago when I climbed on the Nordic Track and decided she would get me through thirty minutes of the most boring form of exercise ever known. She calls her chapter on "Motherhood and Daughterhood" the "core" of the book. "It is hard to write about my own mother," she admits. "Whatever I do write, it is my own story I am telling, my version of the past. If she were to tell her own story other landscapes would be revealed. In my landscape or hers, there would be old, smoldering patches of deep-burning anger."

She writes a lot about the wounds passed on from mother to daughter—especially from mothers to firstborn daughters. Part of me really wants a girl. I think I'd like to raise a daughter who learns how to feel her feelings when she's in them, who learns how to recognize what she wants and how to ask for it, who can separate from her mother without creating alienation for either her mother or herself. Yet another part of me—the part that knows that badly conducted mother-daughter separations go way back in my maternal line—is scared shitless that it won't be a boy. Well, whatever sex it is now, it's not up to me, and it's not going to change. I just have to wait for the twenty-week sonogram that will tell me what my work for the next twenty years is going to be.

I have no idea how to write about how I feel about Mom. Here's what I know: we're about as close as two human beings can be—after all, I was the one who made her a mother. I was the first one to come from her body; she raised me; we were best friends till I was about fourteen. I feel closer to her than to almost any human being in the world. I know her tastes and desires intimately: the foods she likes to eat, the books she likes to read, the clothes and jewelry she likes to wear. I know to buy her turtlenecks because her neck and wrists chill easily; I know to buy her earrings with solid-gold posts or wires because of her allergic reaction to baser metals. She's my origin, the place I come from, the place I go back to. Her eyes, her voice, and the scent of her skin are the most familiar stimulants to my senses. This is how I know she gave me, as an infant, what she herself had been denied: the cuddles, the gaze, the wonder.

Yet we're so far apart. I was the baby who turned her life upside-down. I'm the one of her three children whose life looks least like hers. When my hormones kicked in, we fought like cats sometimes, and that didn't stop for ten or twelve years. I was the adult child with whose opinions she most disagreed. I will probably put my child into day care: how could I put my child into *day care?* — after all the times I heard Mom rail about the "selfish" women who wouldn't give up their own lives for their kids, the "greedy" families who wouldn't curb their material desires — as she had, so stringently — to live on one income?

I love her more than I can express, in ways that I can't express.

I don't want to be like her as a mother — not totally.

What a relief to admit these things. It also feels like a betrayal. She always wants to be perfect at everything — even mothering. I learned from her to place this demand on myself. But no one can be perfect.

Maybe this is a bottom line I can count on with my own child, whether it's a boy or a girl: no matter how much we fight, no matter how we disagree and move away from each other, a closeness will always remain. An indestructible closeness, as ineradicable as the scent of my own skin.

Walked with Luisa again last night. She looks great but is unhappy because she can no longer do her four-mile lunchtime run. Last night we walked to the bookstore, but halfway up the steep hill we had to stop because Luisa couldn't breathe. I feel bad for her because she has always run to keep fit. I'm nearly sixteen weeks pregnant, and like her, I can't handle that much bouncing in my breasts and my belly. I have the sensation that my uterus is hung between two strong guylines inside me and doesn't like to be tugged at.

Wanted to write early this morning; it's 8:30 now and I've been up two hours; but my head aches and I'm trying to decide whether to take one pill now or more later. I've been feeling that tired ache in my body, the way it gets before a migraine knocks me down; also the confusion, the transposing of letters when I write, the transposing of syllables when I speak, dropping things, tripping, not lifting my feet high enough on the stairs.

We've decided to have our baby at a birth center run by a group of six midwives. We visited the two midwifery groups in town and decided to go with this one, even though the other group's facilities were in a beautiful Victorian house only a block away. This group of six have

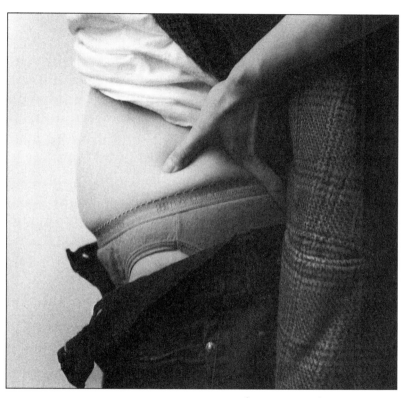

Nineteen weeks pregnant.

between them more than fifty years of experience helping women have babies, and the other group could not match that. I felt a little rude faxing the OB's office and asking them to forward my records, but I feel so much more comfortable with the midwives. Last night we had our four-month prenatal visit with a midwife named Kathy. I expected, since they said she's the center's director, that she would spend the usual fifteen minutes with us as the doctor always did, but she stayed with us for an hour, mostly asking us questions about our feelings about the pregnancy, something the doctors never did. She also encouraged us to ask questions of our own.

She held the Doppler against my belly. She wrote in my records that the top of my uterus is "one-half UB," or halfway to the umbilicus or navel. "Right on target for fifteen and two-sevenths," she said. I'm fifteen and two-sevenths weeks pregnant. The heartbeat was 160 beats per minute, whooshing strong and clear and then diminishing as the little body turned around inside its spaceship. Then suddenly the heartbeat dropped to a slow pounding, half its previous rate. We all leaned forward. Kathy, with her earphones on, probed and listened with a faraway look: *Houston, have we got a problem?* No contact for half a minute. — Static — then that steady whooshing again, with a slower beat in the background: my own heart, that's been beating for thirty-two and five-twelfths years.

"I want it to be OK," I said, settling my head back down on the pillow. Kathy turned to me and said softly, "Of course you do. Maybe it got tangled in the cord. Maybe it grabbed the umbilical cord — though I doubt that because the cord's about as big around as the little body

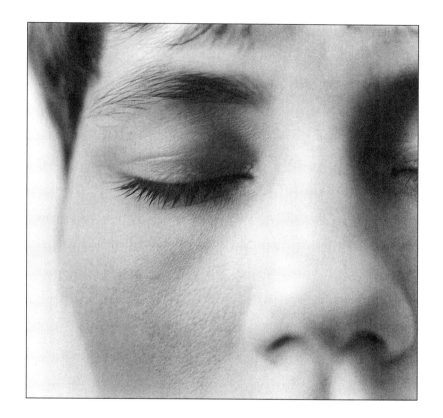

itself," she said. "Maybe it moved and the Doppler picked up only every other heartbeat."

"But is it OK?" I demanded.

"Yeah, probably," Kathy said.

Probably? "I'm *sure* it is," said Nick, who knows the looks of my face and my propensity for worry.

"Look, if you're worried *now,* wait till the baby comes — it only gets *worse!*" Kathy joked. She has two kids.

If it grabbed or got tangled in the cord and that's what caused the heart-rate drop, then it can't do without me, not even for a minute. The cord is connected to the placenta, a big red pancake stuck into the side of my uterus. It is *part* of my uterus, for the time being, in fact: the placenta is its own organ, but it is so embedded into the wall of my uterus that it can't come off on its own. It needs the hormone oxytocin, which causes it to be shaved off and expelled during labor. Everything I put into my mouth crosses that slim margin, from the capillaries of my uterus into that pancake. It's like cooking: you can't fry a pancake in butter without the pancake absorbing some of the butter. The more butter you use, the more butter soaks into the pancake. So I eat well, whole grains and fresh vegetables, dried fruits for iron, milk and yogurt for calcium to build bones and teeth (even the teeth, I read, are formed before birth as little buds on the jawbone), fruit for dessert. Lots of filtered water. Oranges — "I've never seen you eat an orange," Nick said Sunday after Quaker Meeting when I brought out my fruit snack. Not to mention all the granola, lentils, and organic whole-wheat pasta.

The result is a body so clean inside and out that I have no skin blemishes, my hair is not stringy when I wake in the morning, my fingernails no longer break, I do not even get sniffles. To my amazement, one 30 mg codeine-and-Tylenol kills a headache dead. Before I got pregnant I was taking two 50 mg butalbital—a barbiturate, the first-line treatment these days for chronic daily headache—and following up with another one or two just two hours later, and the headache always came back. Now I feel *guilty* that I take anything at all.

I want my baby to be OK, but still, when the pain starts, I think, then I think twice and then again and again, and I sometimes take a pill. Maybe I'm worrying too much about it. Kathy didn't bat an eyelash when I said I'm taking codeine. While she was examining my pelvis I told her about my fear that I've done something harmful by taking medication. "But you were in pain, right?" she said. "You couldn't have done anything else. You have to survive." How am I ever going to survive after the baby comes if I agonize over every little thing now?

Reading Roiphe's book on mothering "in the modern world." It's full of crass generalizations about mothering and women's experience, but she articulates some of my own feelings, central among them my need for men in my life, specifically the men in my family—my husband, my father, my brother, my father-in-law. The baby will need Nick, and if it's a boy, I believe that primarily Nick will teach him how to be a man.

Roiphe also talks about her inborn biological need to have children. I've never forgotten the dream I had when I was twenty-two of my daughter running to me and flinging her arms around me, my catching her and swinging her around. There are ways of reading the little girl as myself, which I didn't know about at the time. All I know is that on waking I had a visceral knowledge that she was not me—she was my child, and I was her mother. This was the beginning of my desire to have kids. It was driven back underground—or up into my head—when I went to graduate school, when I read Steinem and then studied Brownmiller and Rich, the '70s American feminists and some of the French feminists. I thought of men as the impregnating force and women as the "oppressed," victims to our own unenlightened urges. After all, we kept getting back into bed with the enemy—shouldn't we be able to resist this urge? At the same time as this argument was going on in my head, I was falling passionately in love with a man, and for a long time I wanted little else but the feel of his chest hair against my breasts, his musky smell on my skin, his husky man's voice, his big hands on me, his body, utterly different from my own, on top of me and underneath me and all around me, inside me.

Even after that desire diminished, I wanted to remake my life with him. I wanted to negotiate the problems of fitting two lives together. To make myself vulnerable by admitting my dependence on him. I need him. I could make it without him—I know if he were to get hit by the proverbial bus this afternoon I could pay the mortgage, handle the bills, maintain my other relationships and my work. The way I need him is that, without him, I'm not exactly myself anymore. If he's taken from me, then I'd have to change again, and become or evolve a self that now doesn't exist, a self shaped this time by grief and loss, memory and courage.

✹

Charlee took pictures of me with my tomato seedlings today. They all came from a friend whose brother sent her the seeds from Bulgaria. In a tiny tomato seed is hidden the genetic programming, like the invisible tracings on a silicon chip, that make the plant grow leaves, pink stem, tiny hairs, and either red, pink, or yellow fruit. It can come in the mail from Bulgaria and grow in our American soil.

I was surprised Lily had given me so few seeds, because she wanted me to try growing them for both of us, but nearly all of them germinated. Fertility: Jeri said, the day I told her I was pregnant, "Well, at least you know your *plumbing* works."

✹

The news just came—Nick has won the university's Chancellor's Distinguished Public Service Award. We're invited to a party at the Chancellor's mansion. I never ask this, but—what the hell am I going to wear? I've made a kind of secret promise with myself that I would never force myself to go to one of those horrible maternity shops, where they charge you three times as much as anywhere else and you can't return anything. I guess it's time to pull out the sewing machine . . .

✹

Since I read Roiphe, I've been rereading certain passages other authors have written about mothering that have stayed with me ten years or more. I've actually got these passages memorized. I've thought about them so often that they've become part of the fabric of the way I think of myself as a writer and a woman—and, soon, a mother.

I read these essays compulsively in part because it feels impossible to talk to my mother about feeling torn between work and being a mother, about wanting a child so much but also feeling that the work of mothering — never-ending, ever-present — threatens my work as a writer. Mom quit working outside the home when she got married. She's one of the most intelligent women I've known, her mind seemed always to be looking for new things to engage it, and yet she never went back to work.

Partly it was what the culture expected in 1963: you get married, you quit your job, you have babies. Partly it was that she didn't care much about the job she quit; she'd always wanted to be a teacher, but her father wouldn't let her go to teaching school. Her father's refusal to support her desire to be a teacher, I think, fractured her self-confidence. She took a secretarial job, the same sort of job her own mother had taken after her mother's family forced her to leave school: history repeating itself. Mom worked her way up to being executive secretary to the head of a branch of a national insurance company. This guy valued her so much, she always told me, that he offered to arrange a transfer for her when she announced her wedding plans. She first told me this story when I was ten or eleven.

"Why didn't you do it, Mom?"

She couldn't drive, she said (another commonplace competency her father denied her). She didn't know Pittsburgh, she said. She's forever bemoaned her bad sense of direction but has seldom tried to improve it. "The office was on Wood Street, way downtown," she said. "I didn't know where Wood Street was. I would never have been able to find it."

At ten or eleven I accepted this explanation and began to imagine what Wood Street must be like. We never went downtown because my mother has always disliked cities, and hates to drive in city traffic. Soon my image of downtown Pittsburgh was a labyrinth filled with New York skyscrapers, Londonesque winding streets, the foreignness of Paris or Prague or Moscow. At twenty, as an intern at a downtown public relations firm, at the top of one of Pittsburgh's dozen or so legit- imate skyscrapers, I looked up at a street sign and found I was standing on Wood Street. A shiver of having crossed some boundary came over my body. There I was, standing in the middle of the river my mother had been afraid to ford, and after all that, it was just a creek. And it hadn't been difficult: I had taken a bus, I had walked, I had, on my lunch hour, gone exploring — something that takes not only curiosity, which my mother has in abundance, but also confidence. Having a work life takes confidence.

I don't think Mom ever lost the desire to be a teacher. She worked fourteen years as a Sunday school teacher; she loved the kids she taught, and planning their lessons was one of her favorite activities. But I always had the sense that one two-hour class a week didn't satisfy her inborn need to teach, and she always felt inferior because she didn't have a degree. At forty-two, the year I was a college sophomore, she enrolled at Pitt; in her first semester, she earned straight A's, and the highest grades in her writing class. After that semester, she dropped out, to the dismay of all of us. "I'd be fifty before I'd ever be ready to get a job," she said, and, "It would just put us into a higher tax bracket," and, "The house is a mess. I'm not getting enough help with the house."

"I made motherhood my career," Mom has said many times, proudly. "And look what I produced: three intelligent, independent children."

I remember watching Mom on her fiftieth birthday, thinking that by then she'd have been at the head of a classroom, finally, teaching.

I'm drawn back again and again to these other women's writings about motherhood. Some of the books are falling apart, I've read them so many times. Reading these women is like getting on the phone with Jeri, who mentors me in my work. It's like drinking from a cup of wisdom about being a woman-writer-mother.

One is a passage from a Didion piece about sitting on a rich woman's "terrace by the sea" on an L.A. afternoon in winter, feeling sad and drinking away the "dread" she had, "because I wanted a baby and did not then have one." That phrase hooked me by the throat when I first read it. Through high school and college, and even through graduate school, my understanding was that women are forced to choose between work and motherhood, especially "art" and motherhood. I'd just assumed a writer with the critical success that Didion enjoys would never have children, much less "want" children. Intellectually I know it's possible for women to have kids and work, and be successful at both; intellectually I know that it can be better for children to see their mother happy, creative, satisfied in her work. But emotionally, I never believed I could raise kids and write without selling somebody out, probably the kids.

Then there's that piece by Anne Tyler where she talks about having to take three years away from writing for each kid—five years off for two kids, in her case. She says that when her kids were babies, the story ideas coagulated in her veins, making her feel useless, until she was afraid she'd never get the juices flowing again. But Tyler says motherhood gave her "more of a self to speak from" and made her take more risks in her writing. Not giving up on her kids made her commit more deeply to herself as well. But her boundaries are severe. She gives no interviews and does no book tours. "I will write my books and raise the children. Anything else just fritters me away." That line has repeated itself to me over the years. I can't imagine saying it to myself because my mother, the only mother I know, gave up *everything* for her children. "I will write my books and raise the children . . ."

How much of my life will I feel I have to give up?

I realize now that I've read these essays over and over to myself because I wanted to answer this question before I got pregnant. *How much do I have to give up?* But here I am, pregnant, and I still can't answer it. As it turns out, I can't find my own way without having a child of my own.

Had dinner at Lynn and Jeff's last night with Catherine and Fiona, and I kept catching people glancing at my belly. I felt somehow trapped behind glass, not quite part of the company. "You're pregnant?" Fiona exclaimed.

It's an Event. At least among those in this writers' circle, which includes so few children.

While they're sitting there dazzled by this idea, I'm dazzled by Lynn's diamonds, the solitaires in her ears and the ring — white gold? platinum? — on her left hand. I'm studying their immaculate house, the polished pine floors, the spacious, modern black-and-white kitchen, every surface spotless, the very air apparently dustless, the basketful of guest soaps from around the world the sole elegant decoration in the downstairs powder room. I finger the heavy flatware at their table and remember Helen cautioning me that I can never tell about anyone from their exterior. I have a habit of imagining an entire personality based on one or two details. I look at Lynn, a lithe and gorgeous apparition in black jeans and red knit turtleneck, the scarlet brightening her already brilliant brown eyes. I feel huge. I imagine a wreck, an utter mess, descending upon my own house in September — though I know very well from Charlee's place, where two little girls live, that it doesn't have to be that way.

"Well — at least, not *all* the time," Charlee tells me.

I admitted to Nick today how lonely I feel — how far away from him. I can *tell* him about pregnancy, but he can never feel in his body how it feels to me to have to share the space of my body with another person.

His face was a bit wistful as he listened. "Funny," he said; "I feel lonely in this process as well. At least you have the baby for company." I hadn't thought of that. Maybe because I can't feel it moving yet.

We touch each other tentatively these days, slightly afraid of each other's bodies. Nick's suddenly feels so powerful to me. So does mine. I can feel the blood rushing around in my body, in my belly and between my legs. By six months, the books say, my blood volume will have increased by 50 percent or more, and it's mostly gathered below my waist. When we make love and I can relax past the fear of Nick thinking I'm fat, I become caught up in some kind of hot red tide inside myself. Making love is a real relief.

An interesting session with Charlee yesterday. She brought her daughter Gillian, who had some sort of flu and was throwing up into a towel. Charlee had given her the towel, I guess, because she was throwing up only clear fluid. Initially I was disgusted—a *towel?* As I watched Charlee consoling Gillian through this mess, I realized this is one of the things families have the power to do—they can find ways of dealing with uncontrollable bodily functions. Humane, nonshaming ways of helping each other.

Gillian has startling looks—truly skinny, with huge eyes, an odd shade of green-blue, a pointed chin, and wide high cheekbones, all of which combust in a dramatic manner as unruly and unpredictable as the rest of her personality. Later, zooming to a hair appointment on my bike, I passed their house and saw Charlee's younger daughter, Ally, in her swing on the porch. "You have to meet Ally," Charlee had said. "You'll laugh. She's so different from Gillian." And she was: from fifty paces and at fifteen miles per hour I couldn't see much but her short, stubby little body and chubby cheeks rounding out a stolid expression on her face as she watched me wave.

When Charlee comes to shoot, she gives me advice about art and mothering, but she's so good at doing it that I hardly even notice when it happens. But then I grew up in a household that placed great value on commandments and instruction manuals, which served to explain how to live or to accomplish certain tasks. No wonder the first thing I did when I found out I was pregnant was run out and buy the national bestselling pregnancy instruction manual.

We went to the party for Nick's award last night and ran into David and Joyce. We always love seeing them, but this time it was especially nice because David was the one who nominated Nick and wrote his letter of support. Joyce ran up to me and, in front of everyone (except me) sipping cocktails under the tent at the Chancellor's mansion, she put her hand right on my belly. She drew her hand away, then touched me again and crooned, "It's so beautiful." I didn't know what to say. I felt flattered, but I also felt enormous, like the prize melon. "God, I hope I'm as little as you are when this whole thing is over," I said jocularly. A selfish comment, I guess, but Joyce is lovely. I felt huge, a whale draped in its very own tent of floral-print rayon. I made a swing dress just for the occasion. I don't look good in swing dresses or anything A-line. For that reason I've never made or bought a swing dress. They're designed for the hourglass figure, which I've never possessed—especially now— but they can also accommodate a large belly—"You look great. Really," David said, patting me on the back, and I was not entirely convinced.

Who *cares* how I look, anyway? I try not to care so much how I look, but I feel like a stranger to myself. I can't sleep as I'm used to sleeping, even in my own bed. I can't eat as I'm used to eating. I'm used to running on empty, and pumping in one or two bucks' worth of economy when the engine starts to miss; now my body wants to top up the tank with premium in case I don't make it to the next station.

And whoever it is that's eating all the food has also been poking me lately from the inside out — though I'm not really sure that the little scratchings I feel deep inside come from the kid moving around.

✋

Just came back from the five-month ultrasound. An amazing experience, like looking into a time capsule. Like watching a movie in which divers go down to look inside a ship that's been sunken for years, and the water is dark and murky, and when they shine their infrared lights all you can see are the outlines of things. Spooky and half-blind. It was a bit uncomfortable because I had to have a full bladder — it stabilizes everything and makes the picture clearer.

The nurse slathered my belly with gel and put the curved transducer against my slicked-up skin and right away I could see everything in orange relief — the head, the left ear, the legs, not crossed as they are in all the cartoons in the pregnancy books but knocking at the knees. Like the yoga "child pose," when you've got your shins on the floor, parallel, knees bent, and your upper body draped over your legs. Just as the legs floated upward on the screen and the nurse began to ask if we wanted to know "what flavor" we had, I saw the testicles rise from between the legs and said in a voice that sounded oddly detached even to myself, "Oh—we've got a boy." This surprised her. I guess most people need to have the picture explained to them. She pointed it all out to Nick, who was sitting beside the bed holding my hand.

My son. How many times have I heard Mom say this, with the proprietary swell in her voice? *My son. My SON.*

Nick had wanted a girl. As I watched the picture move on screen, I felt like crying, as though I had let him down which is crazy, because it's not my egg that determines the sex, it's his sperm. I thought of our hike over the weekend in Cook Forest, trying out names and settling on Janina for a girl, because that was a name I had found in the National Archives while researching Grandma's immigration, and trying out the sound of it, *ya-nina,* and various anglicized nicknames— Janine being one, Nina being another. "Nina Coles" sounded nice.

"Well, I guess 'Janina' is out the window," he said, but only a trifle glumly, and when the nurse left to get the doctor I burst into tears and asked him if he was disappointed, and he held my hand and told me that of course he wasn't. He smiled at the screen and at me and I thought maybe he actually would be happy with either a girl or a boy, as he's always said he would be. But even though I was so scared of having a girl, I feel disappointed. How am I ever going to raise a boy? I don't know anything about boys.

It's just a *boy,* for God's sake. It's not as though they said, "You're having an alien."

And then the doctor came in and showed us the stomach, which he said was full, and the bladder, which he said was also full, two good indications that the baby was swallowing well—fetuses, he told us, actually *swallow* the amniotic fluid and pee it out, to get their digestive systems working. He showed us the brain, its various lobes and regions, measuring the head circumference, which was average, like everything else — the femur length, the abdominal circumference, even the heart rate, which at 149 beats per minute was "right smack in the middle of the normal range," between 147 and 151. The doctor was a lanky academic-looking guy with a great sense of humor. He switched the monitor color to magenta to examine the kidneys ("Take a picture of them for me," the nurse said, "I told them you were great at finding kidneys"), then switched it to yellow to find the femurs. The baby will be growing bones for the next three months, then he'll start to put on weight. "I like yellow for bones," he said crisply. "Yellow's a good bone color." And it was. The femurs were already solid enough to appear opaque, like little gold ingots, and when he measured them and plugged the data into the computer software it came up with nineteen weeks, one day, like nearly every other measurement. "Right on target," the nurse said.

Our baby is OK. This pregnancy has been absolutely by the books (not counting all the emergency sections in *Expecting the Worst*). I said to Nick while we were in the waiting room, "Wouldn't it be a scream if this project went smoothly, no complications, a normal labor, and at the end a healthy kid? Wouldn't it be a howl if nothing bad happened?" I can hardly imagine it. Yet each day, one day at a time, nothing goes wrong. "A lovely heart," the doctor observed, enlarging the image on the monitor, pointing out all the chambers and listening to its pulsing. "A really excellent heart. Look at that heart — isn't it beautiful?" he asked the nurse. "It certainly is," she said obligingly. Then he focused in on the penis, pinned the electronic calipers onto each end, and took the measurement. "Eight-point-five millimeters," he said, holding his thumb half an inch away from his forefinger and looking at Nick, adding good-naturedly, "A big one!" I'd better get used to willie jokes. I guess all Real Guys have to bond in this way. He stood up and turned the machine off. "On that note . . . ," I said, and he laughed. He shook our hands, smiled at us in a way the other OBs never had — in short, as though we were real people — and patted me on the foot. "We got a very clear picture, and everything looks wonderful," he said. A tape I replay over and over in my head. "Congratulations."

All the way home I felt like laughing. I did laugh at times. I felt like telling everyone, "I just found out I'm going to have a boy." I told the woman working behind the counter at the photo shop downtown. She looked to me like she couldn't give a damn about kids of any kind — she was in her early twenties, with no makeup and long Janis Joplin hair and chunky silver rings on nearly every finger. The photo shop is always full of artists with John Lennon–style wire-rimmed glasses, or people in unpressed oxford shirts and high-top sneakers, or women with dark red-brown lipstick or no makeup at all. I felt like I fit in all right, disguised in Nick's black jeans and a big white T-shirt, my uniform these days. And as she put the receipt in front of me to sign, I said, "I just found out I'm going to have a boy." I thought maybe she'd mutter disinterested good wishes, but her face broke out into a huge smile, and she exclaimed her congratulations as I stepped into the elevator.

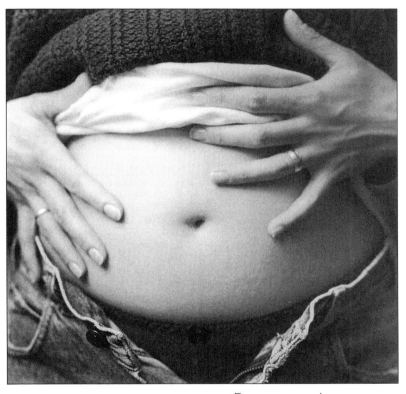

Twenty-one weeks pregnant.

Later, I went to the supermarket to get dinner and as I was picking out some lowfat cottage cheese, reading the labels like I always do now, a little boy approached the case to my right and said in a high, pleading voice, "Mommy, can we get some of these?" He was clutching a six-pack of yogurt marketed to little kids, with cartoon animals all over the pots' labels.

"No," his mother said. "The last time we got those we had to throw every single one of them away. You wouldn't eat them."

"I'll eat them *today*," he said, pleading. I found myself trying to suppress laughter. He was about three and a half feet tall and brown-haired, with a Beatles haircut and a navy blue sweatsuit on. His mother was pretty young herself, certainly younger than I, and she had a baby girl sitting in the food basket.

"Oh yeah, I'm *sure* you'll eat them today," she said, cocking a twisted grin.

"I *promise*," he said, and I laughed out loud.

She looked at me. "I just found out I'm going to have a boy," I said, wishing stupidly that I could get that loop of tape disconnected from my mouth.

"Really?" she said. "Well, don't ever buy him those little tiny yogurts. He'll never eat them."

It was only after I had the lasagna noodles cooked and the spinach stemmed, washed, steamed, and mixed into the cheese that I realized lasagna doesn't call for cottage cheese — it calls for ricotta. Seeing the baby, his brain, his heart, his bones, short-circuited my wires for the rest of the day. He really is there, I kept thinking. He's there. He's real.

Sent my slides off to the graphic design workshop in August in Maine. In the nick of time, thanks to second-day air. If I'm accepted, I'll be eight months pregnant when I go. How big will I be at eight months? — I have no idea. Momentarily it occurred to me that maybe I shouldn't go to Maine this year. It's bound to be uncomfortable, but if I stop doing stuff because of a kid before he's even born, I feel like it will be the first step on the slippery slope of giving up everything I want for the rest of my life. Why not take him to Maine? I can at least try.

Had coffee with a friend who's soon moving out of town. It's clear that she's moving away from her boyfriend. We talked for a while about her plans, but she kept asking questions about my pregnancy. The conversation would veer off toward work, hers or mine, and she would bring it back with a shy question — had I begun eating differently? — what was it like to be pregnant? I talked about the stuff I've learned. How the blood volume increases by half. The midwife's advice to build my hemoglobin with iron-rich foods. How the hormones expand the ribcage even before any organs are shifted into that space, making breathing more of a chore. How, when I come downstairs in the morning, I feel like I could eat everything in the kitchen pantry. How I've kept exercising, taking bike rides and long walks and doing heavy gardening. How the same hormones make the joints relax and the body feels more flexible than ever.

Finally I asked her about her desire to have children, which we'd discussed some time ago. Her boyfriend has an adult child from a previous marriage, and she said he apparently doesn't want a baby at this time in his life—"That's just not in his realm." She talked about an uncle of hers who stayed with his wife after discovering she never wanted children, and now he's filled with regret. As she talked, a veil seemed to drop from her face, and I saw that she's the kind of woman I wish I could be—the kind who would plan to have a kid by going off the pill or ditching her diaphragm, charting her temperature to determine when she's ovulating, then enjoying the process of "trying" with her husband or partner. Oh—and of course, being unequivocally thrilled to see two lines show up on her home test. Maybe she didn't think so, but it wasn't just she who envied me; I was envying her as well.

❦

Judy and Tim are having a girl! They had their ultrasound last week. (Luisa has had two ultrasounds, but the baby crossed its legs both times and wouldn't budge even when the nurse poked at it through Luisa's belly, so she's probably not going to know till it comes.) Physically, Judy's not doing well. She has nonstop heartburn and has begun to throw up—not a good experience in the second trimester. She says Tim doesn't know what's the matter. And emotionally—well, she might be having all the feelings I'm having, but she's not talking about them as much as Luisa and I do. Which is just her personality: she's more practical than I am, always has been. She's a chemical engineer, after all. She told me one thing today, though: that before she got pregnant she was dreaming of babies "nearly every night," but since her pregnancy test she's had only one baby dream. I think she's a little bit frightened—as we all are (sometimes I'm more than a little bit). "I'm still a kid in my mind," she said. "In my head, I'm still seventeen.

I just feel like, when I have a kid, I'll never be able to be a kid myself anymore."

I think my marriage to Nick did this for me. It was the decision to marry him, and then carrying it out in the Quaker manner that we chose, that made me leave behind my adolescence. I went through so many feelings of "leaving childish ways behind" at that time that the process of having a child feels more to me like a deepening of adulthood. For me, it's like going farther into the forest, not entering it for the first time.

Did a full day's gardening today. Spent the morning planting seeds for annuals — nicotiana, four-o'clocks, cosmos. Then put in a climbing rose near the front porch and some stock seedlings. Each time I sit, the baby seems to stand up. Finally this morning I took one pill because my head still hurt, and he didn't kick for about three hours. This upsets me — not to have him move around.

Sometimes I sit watching my bare belly and I can see him moving from the outside. When I first saw my belly undulating, I didn't feel wild joy from what the books call "quickening." I was just startled. I felt the copper taste in my mouth, the way I feel when I get scared or shocked. I'm overwhelmed by feelings of protection. It's not at all a thought in my brain; it's cellular. It's an appetite, like wanting to eat. I want to make sure he can move. I want to make sure he's healthy and happy.

We ran into a poet friend tonight at the Greek food festival. She was on her own — her husband is doing research in Germany for another month and "he's been calling me from every German truck stop," she said. After some small talk I asked her if their decision not to have kids was connected to her commitment to her writing. I told her I'd understand if the question was too personal and she didn't want to answer.

She said she had a miscarriage. She said that she'd become pregnant as I had, in a not-exactly-planned way. She decided she wanted to have the baby, but she miscarried at the end of the first trimester. This was seven years ago. I don't think she told many people. She said she took it hard. She said she and her husband talked about whether they would try to have another child, and "I think we just decided that we wouldn't — that we would have another kind of life," she said.

She said she hadn't wanted kids until actually becoming pregnant, and that she'd been very sick those three months. What astonished her about pregnancy making her so sick was the rebelliousness of the other being inside her. "As women, we like so much to be in control of our bodies, but so often we have to give that up," she said. "It's like your body doubles, there's someone with you all the time. And you can wake up in the morning and think, 'OK — I'm *hungry!*' And the pregnancy tells you, 'Oh, no, we're not — I think we're going to *throw up* for the rest of the day!'"

We sat, the three of us, listening to the Greek band and watching the kids perform intricate Greek dances, and her face was full of color the entire evening, as though she had spent too much time in the sun over the weekend, but there were moments I thought I saw her eyes fill with tears.

Charlee came over for a shoot today. We spend more and more time talking these days while she's taking pictures. It's not small talk; we're becoming good friends. Today we talked about her feelings about not being able to have biological children. She brought it up. She said a friend of hers asked her if it made her envious or upset to look at my belly week after week.

There have been many occasions that it has crossed my mind to ask Charlee about her feelings. I'm not sure why I haven't. Maybe because I've heard so much about how emotionally devastating infertility can be. I'm curious about her feelings but don't want to bring up a subject that might hurt to talk about. So I brush off the few questions that have crossed my mind: "I wonder how Charlee feels about framing my belly in her viewfinder?" "I wonder how Charlee's going to feel when she reads about my ambivalence about being pregnant, about my hostility toward my expanding belly?" One adoptive mother I interviewed for my work with Jeri told me she decided to adopt because she was so tired of blaming herself for her inability to get pregnant. She was exhausted from the succession of medical tests that reinforced her sense of having failed, not only at a desired project but as a woman. For her, deciding to adopt a child was a freeing choice. "It was liberating to make the choice not to keep trying to get pregnant," she said. "My belief to the core of my being is that Alex was meant to be our child. Our own bodies couldn't get him here. This was the way he came to us."

Charlee feels the same about her girls. She says she told her friend it never occurred to her to be jealous, because she has two kids of her own. Her daughters are her own as much as my kid will ever be "mine." "I just didn't have the experience of pregnancy—that's all," Charlee said.

♥

Went to see *Some Mother's Son* this evening. The plot was about the violence of the British government and the IRA, but I was thinking about the title and watching the gender politics play out. *Some Mother's Son* suggests to me that the film's focus is gender politics, not the war. It was produced by Helen Mirren, who played the mother of one of the hunger strikers. I found myself in tears at the beginning, when she takes her family to a village Christmas Eve party and asks her son to dance with her because she wants to dance with "the best-looking man in the room." He throws her a saucy smile and says, "Well, I dunno, Ma, I guess you'll have to make do with me," and he swings her around. Even at this early point we know he will wind up in prison trying to starve himself to death and she will have to watch him do it, but her character doesn't know any of this yet. She just tells him she has forgotten how tall he is and looks up into his face and says, "You remind me so much of your father," who has died, we don't know how, but presumably as part of "the Troubles," and just then I was swept away by the sadness of life (and probably by my hormones)—of daring to bring a child into the world and take care of him so he can grow up and do things he may believe in but I may not. And loving him the entire time. I don't even know who this kid is but already I sense the depth of the sea I'm wading into, and the strength of its undertow. I will raise him so that he can be drafted, maybe. And maybe to resist the draft, be a conscientious objector — or maybe not. Ultimately I'll raise him so he can leave me and live his own life, and sooner or later — but eventually — die. The only thing that makes it possible for me to keep on doing what I'm doing is to look only at what I have to do today, and to ask the stars for strength. I figure if this is what I'm supposed to be doing, then I should have faith that I'll be given strength enough to do it, bit by bit.

For me tonight, this film was an exploration of the separation between mother and son, and the lasting bond. At the end she decides to save his life by putting him on life support. Which is exactly what he begged her *not* to do. But we see her looking at his comatose, ulcerated, starved face and know that she knows *her* decision is separate from his. And she makes hers for herself, not for him.

Nick was complaining that I complained too much this evening. (We went to a bar after the movie — the music was too loud to hold a conversation, and the air was so smoky I felt like a side of ham within five minutes.) I reminded him he always said I'd be "a bear" if I ever got pregnant, and that I think I've been pretty good so far.

"Am I supposed to be *grateful* for that?" he shouted.

"Yes! *I am,*" I shouted back. "I could be complaining all the time — not just some of the time. I don't have my body anymore, I don't have my clothes anymore, I don't have my own sleep anymore, I don't even have my own pee—I'm peeing for somebody else every ninety minutes. I'm totally out of control practically every minute of every day."

I stood in the kitchen, squawking like a bluejay and flapping my arms; he broke into a laugh and relented.

✋

We had a Mother's Day dinner a night early at my grandmother's last night. Judy and Tim came down from Cleveland, and Joe and Claudine were there too. Seeing my brother these days makes me aware in a new way how very difficult it must have been for Mom to have gotten pregnant—accidentally—with Joe just two months after she had me, and at age twenty-three.

Judy's really roughing it. She has chronic heartburn and constant headache and carries economy-size bottles of Rolaids and Tylenol in her purse. Pregnancy, she says, does not agree with her. She doesn't need to say it—you can tell just by how pale she is. I'm sure that after she has the baby she'll get back to volleyball and regain her energetic appearance, but right now she looks uncomfortable.

I wonder what it is that makes two genetically related people respond so physically differently to pregnancy. Even before we got pregnant Judy was already five or six inches taller than I, but now she looks a lot more "pregnant" than I do. She's retaining a lot of water; her breasts and belly were pushing at the fabric of her jumper. These days I usually feel enormous, but last night, walking beside her, I felt as though I didn't "show" at all. That feeling has stayed with me all morning and into this afternoon, and now I'm wondering if something's wrong with me or if I am eating incorrectly. Maybe the kid isn't getting enough to eat? — but the sonogram said he was totally on target in all his measurements! I'm still only 128 pounds and the ultrasound was nearly two weeks ago, so I haven't put on any weight in two weeks? — soon, though, I will be 129. The scale keeps hovering nearly there.

Jesus, I'm watching the scale "hover." I'm really neurotic about this "fat" thing. I know it comes from being fat as a kid. Rolls of fat around my belly; the other kids constantly making fun of me; never feeling normal or acceptable.

Either I feel too fat, or I feel too thin. Maybe, just maybe, for once, I'm just right.

We passed the still shots from our ultrasounds around. Mine were two large color shots and Judy's were tiny black-and-white pictures. It was very difficult to distinguish anything in her pictures. Ours are very clear — even Tim says so. Mom wanted me to point out everything in the picture. My grandmother did too — she kept looking for the penis and seemed real disappointed that it wasn't featured in the still shot. Then the pictures came to Joe, who studied the machine's specifications printed on them and began grilling Tim about the ultrasound's power in megahertz and the technology of its resolution.

"How can it be a cross section and still look so three-dimensional?" he demanded of Tim, who pleaded ignorance about the mechanical aspects.

"Once you get into hertz, I'm no longer an engineer, I'm just a doctor," Tim said.

"But I thought you *were* an engineer," Joe countered — in fact, Tim's bachelor's degree is in engineering — then remembered this was supposed to be a party and decided to lighten up.

Nobody in the family asks any questions about the details of the pregnancies and the things we imagine for our kids, the way everyone at Meeting and all our friends do. No discussion of how we'll handle winter semester in England next year, no curiosity about cribs or clothes, methods of delivery or feelings about becoming a mother. And this dinner was for Mother's Day. No marvelling — as I do — at the fact that, as mothers-to-be, we can feel our kids moving around inside our bodies.

Nick actually gave me a card this morning, and a CD as a present. The card is huge and pink, embossed with flowers, and has a lacy kind of trellis glued on the front. "Did you notice the sparkly bits behind the lace?" he said with a smirk. I guess he spent a while picking it out. I hope the kid inherits his sense of humor.

We made love in the shower this morning. In seven years of being together, we never made love in the shower except for that time last Christmas. The feeling this morning was so spontaneous and reminiscent that I told him I felt sure that's where this kid was conceived. In the shower.

A Quaker friend of ours couldn't help but squeeze and touch me today after Meeting. She kept hugging me, telling me I'm beautiful. Just as Nick asked to speak with her regarding some committee concern, she said, "In a minute; but first, I have to ask your wife to let me feel this belly." I let her. Why do people want to touch it? — for some people the desire is irresistible, like petting a kitten or a teddy bear. She ran her manicured hand over the bulge of my skirt. I was wearing my red lawn dress, made from the fabric I found at Liberty in Oxford Street last year. She cooed, "Ooooh, it's so *beautiful!* You're so demure and small." I still haven't gotten used to thinking of myself as small. In fact I am not small — I'm wearing a 38 bra. That is not small. I am larger than I look. I have broad shoulders and a strong, wide back — all those Slavic genes. And I'm certainly nowhere near being *demure.* At the same time as I'm thinking how inaccurate her description of me is, I'm also thinking that I'd better store up the pleasure of all this attention — after the baby comes, it will all be for him.

Cruised the garage sales yesterday looking for a crib. It was a dreary May day, never getting above 45 degrees. I showed up at 8:35 for a sale advertised for 9:00, figuring it would be open a few minutes early. The woman who came out to meet the small crowd gathered on her doorstep looked to be in her late thirties and was adamant that we had to wait outside in the rain until 9:00. I stood with two old ladies, both under five feet tall. One of them asked the owner if there was a stroller, and the owner said the woman would have to wait and see what it was like. I asked the owner to tell me about the crib. Her face softened then, and she said, "It's beautiful."

"How much do you want for it?" I asked.

A line appeared on her forehead and she told me I'd have to wait and see. "Oh, come on!" I protested, but she went back into the house and bolted the door.

The old ladies and I began to chat. They wanted to know how much second-hand stuff I was buying. "My son, everything he buys has to be new," one of them said. She was the grandma—the other one was her sister. There were three grandchildren, all boys. I said I couldn't afford all new stuff. "Neither can he, believe me, honey," the grandma said. Her sister was narrowly inspecting my clothes—Nick's black jeans, my down overcoat, and the leather clogs I bought last summer in Maine.

"What country are you from, honey?" she said.

I opened my mouth to respond but was so surprised that nothing came out, and I just stood there in the drizzle with my jaw hanging open. What *country* was I from?

"Are you American?" she said.

I managed to answer that. "I was just looking at your shoes," she explained. "They look like something that someone from a foreign country would wear."

When we finally got into the garage, the crib looked pretty nice. Nick says he wants to buy a new crib because babies chew on cribs. "You'll never find a used crib without gashes and bites on the railings, and peeling paint," he said. This crib was made of a light varnished hardwood, maybe maple, and its corners were curved. It looked like a piece of real furniture, like a bed frame you might buy for yourself, except extra-small. I looked for teeth marks and couldn't find any. Nick had mentioned that some cribs came with plastic strips across the railings that prevented a baby from biting the wood, and I saw that this crib had those. They didn't even seem to have been bitten. But when I tried to lower the railings they didn't go down easily, and I noticed there was a bit of rust on some of the metal works, and there were some cracks in the vinyl cover on the mattress. I asked the owner how old the thing was. "Fifteen years," she said immediately. A fifteen-year-old crib, and she was asking ninety dollars? I could probably pay less than double that for a new crib, though I didn't know for sure because I hadn't shopped around. For a minute I wished I had Nick with me because he'd used cribs before and knew what to look for. It seemed shaky. And one railing didn't seem to want to stay up, which the owner blamed on the uneven surface of her garage floor.

I asked the grandma under my breath what she thought. She poked at the mattress and peered at the wood and tried one of the railings, finally pursing her mouth and saying, "Well, honey, I'll tell you — I got my daughter a crib like this for twenty-five dollars and it was top of the line, beautiful, untouched, and it came with everything. This here, I don't know, it's up to you," and she walked away, shaking her head ominously. It didn't look that bad to me, though. I felt like Linus looking at Charlie Brown's little Christmas tree — "All it needs is a little love." But it was so old. "How much will you come down?" I asked the owner. "Make me an offer," she said tersely. Half of ninety was forty-five, so I said that I didn't think I would pay more than fifty dollars for a crib this old. She nearly snorted and said no. So I gave her my card, told her to call me if it hadn't sold by the end of the day, and wished her good luck.

In the evening, she called back and left a message saying that her name was Ruth and that she'd sell me the crib for fifty dollars, and to call her back. Cheapskate that I am, right away I wished I'd said forty dollars, or something lower. I should have known no one would take it. I told Nick it was old and seemed a little shaky and one railing wouldn't stay up. I told him what the grandma had found for her daughter and that we could probably find something better at a better price. I decided to let it go.

But this morning Ruth called again. I tried to put her off, saying I was worried the slats were too far apart, against federal guidelines. People had told me to be careful to pick out a crib with slats no more than two and a half inches apart, or the baby's head might get stuck between them. I never would have thought of that. How big is a baby's head, anyway? She was very polite in the face of this transparently bullshit excuse and said everything was up to code, that she and her husband had checked it out the previous evening. I tried to get out of it but wound up making an appointment for this afternoon.

So Nick and I drove up the hill. The crib had been set on level concrete, and the railings worked on the level. Smoothly, in fact. Without a crowd of people around picking over the baby stuff like vultures, this crib looked like a very nice place for our kid to sleep. She said she had bought it at Babyland, the city's best-known baby store. She and her husband had found the serial number when they turned it upside down, and the last numbers were 83, showing it had been purchased in 1983, in case we ever needed to contact the manufacturer, which was Child Craft. Nick liked it. Everything worked well, and Ruth had put the wheels on. She was very solicitous and hovered around, showing us how to work the various parts and said she would get her husband to demonstrate how to dismantle and rebuild it.

So we said we'd buy it. Nick went to pull the car around to the alley in back of the house. I asked her if they were moving, or what. She glanced around—the playpen had not been taken, either, and there was an old brown-plaid carriage—and she grasped her elbows, saying, "No, it was just *time.* "

"Time to clear things out?" I said. She was a thin, attractive woman of medium height, with permed light-brown hair cut to chin length and light brown eyes, and as I watched her face she gestured mutely toward the playpen and the crib. "Time to get rid of the baby stuff?" I said.

"It's *hard* to do this," she said with a strained smile.

"Hard to sell the crib?" I said.

She sighed. "When I look at this crib, I think of my elder son. He's fourteen. He slept in this crib, and then his brother after him. And I always thought that number three would come," she said, her smile turning a bit wistful. "But it never did. And—if I were going to have more children, let's face it, I shouldn't be selling this stuff, right?

"And I think about it now—I'm forty-one," she said. "That's getting old. Do I really want to have another kid *now?* " Evidently not. She had just remodeled her kitchen, she said—all those brand-new cabinets just waiting to be scuffed and banged up by a toddler. Her older son was getting ready for high school next year. So the crib was being passed to another person who could use it.

We took it apart and stacked it carefully in the car. Her husband did come down to teach us the dismantling. "Wait!" she called when she saw me stacking the railings on top of the springs. "The springs are the thing that scratches everything else." She gave me plastic bags to layer in between. We chatted a while about schools and the new superintendent and the inadequacy of city kindergartens, the late afternoon sun shining into our eyes, and she told me that, for Mother's Day, her kids had made her breakfast in bed ("That's *de rigeur,*" she said. "Is it?" I asked), and she commented how appropriate it seemed to buy a crib on Mother's Day. Then I gave her the check and we drove away.

Went for a walk with Luisa last night. Six weeks ago when we took our first walk, we said we were going to do this every week, but the weather's been horrible.

It's so pleasant talking about pregnancy with her.

I had to ring the bell twice at Luisa's house. She was in the bathroom. "You know the *problems* I've been having," she said. Constipation is common in pregnancy. The books all say you should avoid it as early in the pregnancy as possible or all kinds of things result, hemorrhoids being the most unpleasant and persistent among them. Luisa says she's tried every remedy from Metamucil to Senokot. What she hasn't tried is plain old food and water. She listed for me all the food she ate yesterday.

"You're missing your fresh vegetables," I said.

"I have vegetable-itis," she said with a grimace. "I don't want to eat vegetables."

"Vegetables doesn't mean broccoli boiled to death, Luise," I said. I told her about the curried lentil soup with carrots Nick had made the previous night, the salad of baby spinach, the enchiladas I invented with julienned squash, onions, peppers, and tomatoes mixed with fat-free refried beans and cilantro. "That sounds *great*," she said.

I also told her how constipation made me get rid of my prenatal vitamins, which are loaded with iron. The iron in supplements isn't absorbed as completely as the iron in food, so a lot of it stays in the guts, where it blocks everything up. When we went to Phoenix I'd thrown a handful of big, white prenatal vitamin pills loose in my toiletries bag. When I opened the bag one morning I found a black, muddy jelly at the bottom. A couple of the vitamin pills accidentally got soaked with saline solution for my contacts. I couldn't believe I'd actually *eaten* that crap. It looked like the black stuff that clogs the drain in the bathroom sink. I promised myself I wouldn't have to eat them anymore.

People are surprised when I tell them I don't take vitamins regularly. It bugs my friends and bugs Nick. (The OB I used to go to told me the prenatal vitamins he prescribed have folic acid to prevent spinal defects, but I searched the Web and found out that folic acid only prevents spina bifida in the month *before* conception. It does something to the immature eggs before they're released. Folic acid after conception is pretty useless against spinal defects.) There's only one book I've found — *Our Bodies, Ourselves* — that says you don't have to take vitamins when you're pregnant. It says you can take any multivitamin, or you can get nutrients from — get this — *food*. What a radical idea. The body, it says, absorbs vitamins better from food than from a pill, because the body was designed uniquely to eat food, not pills. You have to be careful what you eat, of course, but even if you're not pregnant you ought to eat a balanced diet. The midwives were OK with my not taking a vitamin. The midwife told me I should make sure I get iron, because it helps your red blood cells meet the increased need for oxygen, thereby keeping your energy up, but she said getting iron through food is no problem. "You don't have to eat liver," she said. I told Luisa what the midwife told me — eat iron-fortified cereal with dried fruit on top.

Then I told her about my bran solution. Luisa was the one who had told me to read *Our Bodies, Ourselves,* and that's where I learned that the solution to constipation is bran, bran, bran, with lots of water and exercise. I wasn't eight weeks pregnant when I went out and bought a jar of bran. "Bran is what horses eat!" I told her. "Look at their muscles. And their fertilizer." Luisa grimaced again. Two tablespoons of bran go on my cereal each morning. I have a huge bowl of cereal, three different kinds, with lots of fresh and dried fruit and this lowfat milk I get at the supermarket that has yogurt culture in it. The carton says it's "Happy Milk." It puts me in a great mood. My morning cereal is the best thing about my day. I think I should have been eating this way all along; I feel so good. Most evenings, even if I'm not hungry, I also eat a "fiber nightcap," a small bowl of cereal with just one table-spoon of bran.

"Tablespoon?" Luisa said.

"A coffee scoop," I said.

Her lip curled. "And you're regular?" she demanded.

I said, with the vegetables and fruits, the bran and the water, at least four to five days a week I am. This convinced her. I bought her a jar of bran on the way back to her house.

She mentioned she doesn't drink eight glasses of water a day, the way all the books tell you to do. "The bran won't work without it," I said.

"I'm just so tired of peeing all the time," she said.

Judy says she only has to get up once a night to pee. Luisa says she gets up five times. Lately I've been getting up two and three times, always at 1:30 and 3:30 on the dot. It feels like I'm going to pee so much that the toilet will run over, but it's always only about eight drops. Some nights, I told Luisa, I wake from dreams that I'm peeing because I feel the need to pee so badly. "But it's only eight drops!" she said, nodding and laughing.

It's so great to bitch and moan with other pregnant women. *"You will need other women,"* Our Bodies, Ourselves says about pregnancy. "If you don't know any other women who are pregnant, put up a sign at the market or laundromat. *Women were never meant to go through childbearing alone."*

There are all kinds of things Luisa and I ask each other. Do your breasts hurt? Are you hornier than you used to be?

"Do you feel movement all the time?" Luisa demanded last night, like a prosecutor.

"No," I said.

"Do you worry when you *don't* feel it?" she demanded.

"Yes," I said, the docile witness, "when it doesn't move for a long time, I think I've killed it."

"OK," she sighed, "I just wanted to know."

My conversations with Judy are different. "Do you get out of breath?" I ask her. "Do you feel a lot of movement? What does it feel like?" Judy's always matter-of-fact about these things, and her answers are usually short and sweet. She has feelings, but she doesn't focus on them as much as I do. And then, her pregnancy is so unpleasant—constant heartburn, some vomiting, swelling, physical distortion. She does not like being pregnant. It's no wonder she doesn't want to focus on her feelings about it.

When I see myself, I'm no longer surprised by what I see. I see myself, only with a big belly. I look at myself all the time, though; maybe that's why it's not surprising that my own changed image doesn't shock me. Or maybe it's because of the photographs Charlee is taking. Each week she brings me a new set of contact sheets, three or four or five dozen new pictures—all of me. It takes me outside of myself, and I can see what other people see. What I see is the woman in the pictures looking increasingly relaxed and happy with each week that rolls by.

The interior changes are maybe even more dramatic, but they don't surprise me, either. I welcome them and, even more strangely, I've come to expect them. For the first time in my life, I am—and I've become *used* to being—happy and content.

I've been wondering lately about the connection between the body and the feelings. Am I having an "easy" pregnancy in part because of all this written reflection? They say there are studies that show that pregnant women who examine and deal with their feelings about their "changing role" can decrease or prevent pregnancy sickness and compulsive vomiting. As though figuratively "spilling one's guts" heads off the literal response. Studies like this always carry the qualifications that "there is no guarantee" and, essentially, that you can't control anything about pregnancy, no matter what you do. It sounds to me as if a lot of pregnant women are willing to try almost anything during pregnancy to guarantee themselves a shorter and less painful labor. But I don't think anything will guarantee you any outcome in pregnancy. Whether you're expressive, like me, or you're not, like Judy, you're going to get the labor you get, and you're going to have to deal with it.

❦

I've been looking at the contact sheets from our photo shoots. My favorite picture is from when I was sixteen weeks pregnant—a month ago. It's the most honest picture so far. I stand like that all the time, in my real life. In my nonpregnant life, in my pregnant life. In my house. I have bad posture, I slouch, and I always put my hands in my pockets because I don't know what to do with them. And because I don't have to hold them up that way. I'm lazy about how I carry myself. Pregnancy has taught me that. Now I'm bigger, and I have to be more energetic about how I hold my body, how I move around and how I stay still.

From this picture, I can see why people tell me I don't "look" pregnant. The big sweater hides any sign in the midriff. The big pants mask the growth of my belly. It's only from a profile that anyone might tell. And when they find out, they say to me, "Wow — you look *great.* " As though a pregnant woman is supposed to look like — what? the Pillsbury dough-boy? Even the wife of the family doctor we interviewed today said that. "I thought your husband told me you were five months pregnant, but when I saw you walk in I wasn't sure," she said, glancing at my belly, "you look *wonderful.* " In other words, You look *small.* I still have not gotten used to thinking of myself as "small," I was so "big" as a child. I feel comfortable now in my growing body, but I also feel how powerful the ideal of feminine smallness is in the culture, so I'm simultaneously afraid to return and afraid *not* to return to my "pre-pregnancy size," as all the books call it. Of course, I'd like to wear my old size 8 clothes again. But then again, why should I limit myself to the smallest possible body, the smallest possible dress size, when I can look as "wonderful" — as healthy and at home in my own body and my clothes — as I do in this picture?

Woke this morning from a dream in which I had given birth, prematurely and at home but quickly and painlessly, to a little girl — except she wasn't a baby but a toddler almost two years old. She had long, curly, light-brown hair and fair skin — nothing at all like me or Nick.

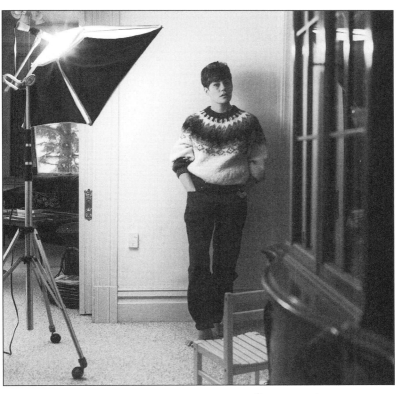

Sixteen weeks pregnant.

And I felt fine and was resting in bed—not our bed and not our house or any house I knew, but I knew in the dream I was "at home." My mother had gone into another room with the baby—in my dream I knew her as "my baby" even though she was so big. Somehow the news came to me that the baby was ill and likely to die. I leaped out of bed—I had my old body back, with no pain—and ran to the kitchen to find my mother and the baby, who was struggling to breathe. I remember I kept thinking, lucidly, "But I was supposed to have a boy," and thought perhaps they'd made a mistake on the ultrasound—perhaps it wasn't a penis we'd seen after all!—but she was dressed in a sage-green sweat-suit and white tennis shoes and she was lying on the kitchen table in front of my mother, struggling to breathe, her back arching to draw in air. My mother was on the phone to a friend from church, ignoring my baby. I picked her up and stroked her hair and she began to calm down in my arms.

"We have to get a doctor!" I said. "We have to get her to the hospital!"

My mother hung up and said, with a baleful expression, "I don't know—she's *very* sick." The phone rang, and rang again, and I asked my mother to pick it up. As though it were an effort, she reached up and got the phone. It was another friend of hers, and her face became animated as she began to chat about some church affair. I dug out the yellow pages with one hand and began looking for an old college friend's number under "Pediatricians," because he is the only pediatrician I know by name, blaming myself because I hadn't yet chosen a baby doctor, my child gasping for breath, my mother on the phone, no help in sight.

"Get off the phone!" I screamed. "We have to get her to the hospital!"

My mother hung up, staring at me. I felt as though it were my fault the baby was sick, and I woke with a certainty that my child would die.

I woke sitting up, my legs hanging over the edge of the bed, crying, in huge loud sobs. It was 6:45 and Nick had been up for an hour preparing a speech, so I was in fact alone in bed. I tried to quiet down because I was afraid our third-floor tenants could hear me, but then I remembered they moved out weeks ago. I cried for a couple of minutes and when I thought I was under control I got up to look for Nick. As I walked down the front stairs I wasn't sure whether I was pregnant — the feeling that I had given birth, had seen the baby come out of me, was still so real and powerful that I thought maybe I was done. But I could still feel my belly and as I saw Nick getting the morning paper from the porch I started to cry all over again, partly in relief and partly in fear because, although the ultrasound was so reassuring, we really don't know anything for certain until the baby's out in the world. I leaned against Nick, crying, and told him I dreamed I'd had the baby and it got sick and died. He held me till I quieted down again.

"What a responsibility you live with every day," he said.

I know the dream's not literal. It represented two extremes of motherhood I'm afraid of — the cool, ultra-rational one and the hysterical, irresponsible one. There were my fears, dramatized: if I express my feelings, I'll be the hysterical mother; if I don't, I'll wind up as the cold mother. There has to be some middle ground.

One of the primary differences between me and Mom is that I say my feelings easily and habitually, and she just doesn't like to. And, unlike me, she planned to get pregnant. I'm organized, but I resist following the example she set of managing and planning everything in advance. Even though it sometimes makes me uncomfortable, I try to invite some spontaneity into my life. I didn't plan to have a baby, and now that I'm having one I'm still not planning for the inevitable problems of his life. He's going to get sick, but I *haven't* chosen a doctor. It's been on my mind to do that.

If I could be that logical mother, I'd have no anxiety about doing our baby any damage through medication or diet because all my faith would be placed in the medical professionals and the rules they set out for me to make a healthy baby. But instead of seeing pregnancy as the process necessary to make a product—a healthy baby—I see it the way I see any relationship. It's mysterious and open-ended. It's not primarily a matter of intellect or logic. For me it's a matter of feelings, and a great deal of any relationship depends on the other person and his or her actions and feelings.

I think the dream is a way of asking myself to reimagine motherhood as a role in the middle ground, one I can fit into, one that will make our baby healthy and happy and me less perpetually anxious and self-critical.

I'm left feeling calm and grateful in the wake of such a scary vision. I think I could sit in this coffeehouse and write for a long time about how grateful I am to be alive, and that the baby's OK.

We all live mostly in a state of getting through the day. We set our alarm clocks and get up on time, we shower and dress, we eat breakfast. We go to work, log on, retrieve our email, our voice-mail, our snail mail. These things have little apparent connection to the larger life we lead — the overall pattern our lives take, the depth of our love for ourselves and each other, our connection to the earth and its life — the things that will carry on after we cease to exist. Our daily consciousness is taken up instead with what to make for dinner, with sending or receiving faxes or FedExes, with meeting deadlines. No mystery to these activities. No apparent mystery to pregnancy, either. For many, maybe, it's a simple cause-effect transaction. Albeit a reason to celebrate — but don't people also celebrate winning the lottery? It's not a lottery. One could see it like that, with the jackpot delivered in nine months. If it's that strictly material, that banal, then why do I have this sense, which envelops me out of the blue, that I'm on a space shuttle? Or the sense that I'm once more falling in love? — or the sense that I'm dying? — these images of journey and passion.

What pregnancy has done is open my senses to ordinary, daily life. Four million American women have babies each year, so pregnancy is one of the most ordinary, everyday occurrences — each day, in America alone, more than ten thousand women discover they're pregnant. In another way, though, pregnancy can be seen as extraordinary — it's a process that only women can carry out. It's something our bodies are uniquely fitted for. Each pregnancy produces at least one singular human being. For this reason, most people pay attention to the physical changes of pregnancy, because they're dramatic and hard to miss, and because they're a direct result of the unique product — the growing baby.

Pregnancy also incurs dramatic psychological and spiritual changes, but they occur so gradually that they can be difficult to notice. It's like any journey. It's like our drive a few months ago from Phoenix to Flagstaff: in the morning we were surrounded by saguaro and ocotillo, and in the afternoon we were deep in snow and fir. If you nap in between, what would you miss? — a lot of sagebrush and scrub on cattle ranches and a high climb — a three-thousand- or four-thousand-foot ascent. Thinning of the atmosphere, a sense of getting on top of the world — the horizon is vast between Phoenix and Flagstaff. There are no hotels there, because the scenery is not the sort that people book a trip for. (Just the same, I can't imagine anyone getting pregnant just to experience what it's like to be pregnant!) But if you pay attention to that part of the journey, you prepare yourself psychically to see the Canyon and its climactic burst of scenery. You prepare yourself to experience it in a fresh way, within its own context, and not as a repeat of the myriad two-dimensional images of it — reduced, cropped, and otherwise defaced — available in the culture. Paying attention to our surroundings during that drive out of the desert and into the mountains, the Canyon made so much more sense to us than postcard images of it ever could.

It's the same with pregnancy. Awareness of the journey has brought me so much more passion than I ever expected. I mean real passion — I mean the feeling of all boundaries coming down, of being dismantled. I've learned that pregnancy is a relationship: a gradual, steady, daily accumulation of information and insight about someone. A desire to satisfy a curiosity you suspect may never be satisfied anyway. It's like marriage. I know more of Nick than does any other person living on the planet. And yet, after knowing him eight years, I could never know enough about him. I could never get tired of knowing more of him. We keep knowing each other in deeper ways. The pregnancy is part of this, too.

What good does it do to try to articulate what is ultimately mysterious? — Here's what I know: after that mother dream, I drove Nick downtown, and I felt as washed out and empty as the streets appeared after last night's rain. I stopped at the Strip to get dinner stuff. As I waited in line to get Nick some Stilton cheese, thinking how much I know he likes Stilton, knees and elbows were going off in all directions in my belly, no longer the questionable scratchings and pokings of two weeks ago but real rumbles. I think they made no mistake that it is a boy — though Judy says her girl does the same thing. Driving home with white, puffy cumulus clouds being pulled across a blue sky by the high winds we've been having lately, I suddenly felt so close to these man-people that have been given to me — Nick, whom I know so well, and this other person, unknown yet, that has been living inside me.

When I see Nick come out of the shower, the cat winding herself around his ankles as she always does in the morning, the reality of his naked body confronts me — the house in which lives the person that has become so dear and so indispensable to me. When he comes home from work and I unbutton the top three buttons of his shirt and inhale the scent of his chest, I wonder who it is living there inside me, and I feel all bound up within Nick's body.

7 A.M. Two weeks have passed since I've been able to bring myself to write in here. A block of some sort.

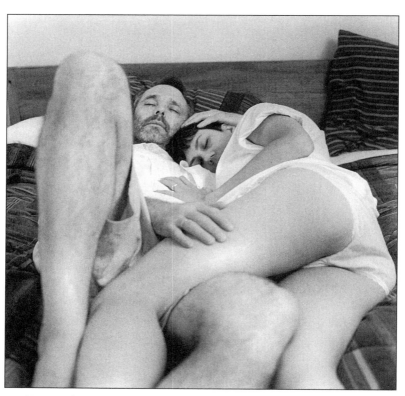

Twenty-five weeks pregnant.

Woke from a dream in which I couldn't leave home. A journey dream. I was going on vacation but I was with my parents and we were driving to Maine, maybe even to England. *Driving* to England? We got ten miles down the road and someone had forgotten something, and even though I hadn't forgotten anything I still felt compelled, in my usual neurotic fashion, to go back into the house anyway, to check my room and rifle through all my stuff, to make sure everything was still there. I had all my own stuff—my green desk, my fountain pen, my leather date book. My beautiful book was coming apart at the seams, though. This grieved me.

Then we drove and drove, and got most of the way there, but suddenly we had come full circle, back to the house, and they were parked in the car waiting for me—my old family, Mom and Dad and Judy (Joe wasn't in the dream)—while I went upstairs to my old room to get something. And I couldn't leave. I remembered I hadn't arranged for anyone to take care of my cat. My baby. I stood crying on the front porch, and shouting, "I can't leave!" Judy shouted back, "Yes, you can!" She gently put her arm around my shoulder and led me to the car.

What would I do without my sister?

But what I forgot to say was that I had also come back to get ink cartridges for my fountain pen. I had forgotten to pack refills so that I could write while I was away. And as I hunted through the desk I couldn't find them. I found green ones, red ones, purple ones that wouldn't fit—not the blue ones I've become accustomed to. Finally, I found them—the ones I'd bought at W. H. Smith's in Leeds.

I couldn't leave home. My book was falling apart. I couldn't write.

I want to be a good mother.

I also want to write. I need to write.

I've stopped writing, and I'm worried.

I've been accepted for the design workshop in Maine. Ken Hiebert is teaching it. Charlee knows a number of people who like his teaching. I'm excited.

Saw Helen last week because I had been so depressed—crying, fearful of writing even in the journal, having all those crazy dreams, unsure of what was happening to me. We talked for a while and she said even though the feelings that had brought me in were melancholy, I seemed to be carrying myself in a relaxed and comfortable way.

She encouraged me not to expect myself to figure out definitively what's going on with me during pregnancy. "You're being shaped so much right now," she said, "that you can't expect to shape yourself too much."

Went for a walk with Luisa the other day. I can't even recall what we talked about, but it was so companionable. We set off in a light drizzle at 9 A.M., and walked down to the bagel shop for a cup of coffee—decaf, of course. She wasn't going to have any of my bagel, but I joked, "I can't bear to have my baby eat without yours eating as well," and she took half. And she poured me some of her coffee.

Ran into Helen outside the post office yesterday. She was with her younger son, a nine- or ten-year-old wearing an oversized yellow polo shirt and khaki shorts way too big for him, the way boys are wearing pants. He was holding her hand. His crew cut made him look like his mother. She was dressed in baggy overalls and a white turtleneck, with bright pink lipstick slashing across her face, and of course she looked wonderful, the way people who are not afraid of their feelings seem to glow and rest easy inside their skin. She was striding down the sidewalk with her little boy in tow.

"I wanted girls," she'd told me last week. "I put in my order for two girls, and didn't get any of what I wanted." But she said, "I love boys, I love having boys," especially "if they have a good father," she said, "because at some point they become like little ducks and go paddling off behind their dads. It's very freeing. Girls are not that way at all. I have nieces and they're always right here," she said, patting her lap, "stuck to me. Boys are like that when they're babies — when you want them to be."

"So you agree with Bly, that men need to be the ones to teach boys how to be men?" I was incredulous. Helen's a strong woman, a feminist for sure; but I should have known she doesn't vote a straight party ticket.

"Absolutely," she said. "It's just the way it is."

Had my teeth cleaned today and the dentist was telling me pregnancy horror stories. Why do some people do that when they know you're pregnant? In the first one, the wife of a friend he knew was two weeks overdue "and never really went into labor," he said. I knew what was coming: she was going to have the baby in some terribly inconvenient place — a bus, a restaurant, standing in the grocery line. I lay in his chair, jaw hanging open, staring into his eyes, which were magnified by two sets of lenses, like twin telescopes, making him look like an owl. He told me this woman called the doctor "because she wasn't feelin' too good one day," and the doctor told her to relax and call him if anything started to happen, so she hung up and went to the bathroom and sat down on the toilet—

I just knew what was coming next.

"—and her water broke, and she screamed for her husband to call 911, and he went and called, and he *swears* he was back in a matter of seconds but by the time he got back he could see the baby. And the paramedics got there in a couple of minutes, but it was too late: by the time they got there she'd already given birth."

"Ungh-huh," I managed.

"That's pretty common," his hygienist said. "You hear stories like that all the time—"

You do?

"—like, women having babies in toilets, or women who don't even know they're pregnant, who are so fat they can't even feel the baby moving. Haven't you ever heard stories like that?"

"Ungh-uh," I said. Earlier, in fact as a way of beginning our "conversation," the hygienist had told me how important it was to floss at least once if not twice every day during pregnancy "because of all the changes in your body, the increased bacteria"—which the dentist later said was caused by "hormones": everything in pregnancy seems to be caused by hormones. "If you don't, you could wind up with *serious problems*," she said. Her eyes glittered through her safety glasses.

"Didn't you ever hear about women losing all their teeth after having babies? — that's what used to happen in the old days," she said.

"Or else you could get these horrible lumps in your mouth called 'pregnancy tumors,' and those don't go away — you have to have them removed; but of course you can't do that until after the baby's born because it's surgery." She merrily described the "pregnancy tumors" as lumps of tissue that grew on both sides of the teeth, were swollen and red and "totally gross. Disgusting." She took her tools out of my mouth and let me rinse.

"Have you ever seen one of these?" I asked, grimacing involuntarily and trying to keep control of my stomach.

"Only in books," she said, adding brightly, "I'll show you." Just then the dentist came in and I asked him if it was really necessary to floss more than once a day, or to take special care of one's teeth during pregnancy. He flipped his face mask off and folded his arms. "Well, you could contract what's known as pregnancy gingivitis — that's when the gums swell, and bleed 'n' bleed 'n' bleed, and when that happens, a lot of times what people will do is they'll quit brushing and flossing, when that's actually the most important thing to do. So it's important to just keep everything as clean as possible. Especially with all the changes in diet: you know, eating different foods—"

But I've only eaten even more wholesome foods since I got pregnant.

" — and snacking all the time—"

What is the image of a pregnant woman, anyway? a pig constantly at the trough?

" — and in general putting food into your mouth more frequently."

What about those pregnancy tumors, I asked. I *had* been feeling a tiny blister on my lip, but it wasn't on my gum—but still—

His double magnifiers honed in to my lip, then he flipped those up, too. "Oh, that's nothing. Probably just a mucus-collecting cyst"—which sounded disgusting enough in itself—"maybe nothing. These tumors are awful, I've seen maybe two in my practice; they don't disappear after pregnancy, you have to have them cut off. Horrible: the women get these big red strawberry tumors. Hormonal: nothing you can do about them."

The hygienist waltzed back in. "Here," she said, and pointed to the page of a book on which was printed a full-color closeup picture of the "strawberry tumor" growing on both sides of the right molar line. The woman's lips seemed to be stretched apart by unseen hooks or clamps. My stomach rolled again. "Oh God," I muttered, thinking distractedly, How could the woman possibly *chew?* And, Why are they showing this to me?

"Isn't it *disgusting?*" the hygienist cried.

"She *loves* that book," the dentist said.

"But look at how bad the teeth are," the hygienist said. "Look at all that plaque and tartar. She probably never brushes or flosses."

"Which is why you should keep on brushing and flossing," the dentist said darkly.

"If I stopped brushing and flossing *today,*" I said, "I still wouldn't wind up like that."

The light above me, and their eyes, shone down into my face. "You *never know,*" the dentist said, only half-joking. "You never know *what* will happen."

Then he proceeded to tell me the story of the guy he knew whose wife gave birth on a back road in the mountains of central Pennsylvania, and he'd had to chew through the umbilical cord. "Here's what happened — and this guy *swears* it was an act of God . . ."

🖐

Judy called around 6 to answer the email I'd sent her last week. She said she and Tim liked my idea of writing about pregnancy.

"Why?" I asked, like a two-year-old.

"I don't know why," she said, "it just sounds interesting. But we thought it would be even more interesting if you had more than one person — if you talked to, like, two or three women instead of just one."

"I do have more than one," I said. "I've got you, and I've got Luisa."

She went wild with disapproval. "Me!" she shouted. "You don't want me! I don't have anything profound to say. All my thoughts are mundane — totally ordinary."

"That's what I want."

"But everything *you* say is — totally *different* from the way I feel," she said. "You're so much more into this whole thing, you're so much more attached. Which surprises me, because I thought I'd be the one who was into it, and you'd be detached."

"Everybody's different," I said. "I think you're going to get attached when the baby's out."

"I know I will," she said.

Everybody is different. It's body biochemistry and emotional constitution. "You've got to do what works for you," Judy said. That's one of the most elementary lessons of pregnancy: your body, which has recently become another person's dwelling place, is changing fast and demands to be listened to, and you have to do not what is good for someone else's body but what is good for your own. It's a highly individual process. Judy throws up, has chronic acid reflux, develops heart arrhythmia (which she had for a few days last week), gains weight over her whole frame. I have no gastric problems and gain weight mostly in my belly, but my thighs and calves erupt in a blistery, itchy rash. Luisa cries every day for four months while I am feeling, for the first time in my life, emotionally balanced.

�

We decided to return the walnut-stained teak and bamboo coffee table we bought last week. Nick really liked its beautiful dark wood, but he said, "If we wanted—ever—to eat dinner in front of the TV, the glass-topped table would be better."

"Or if we wanted to play with blocks, or Matchbox cars, or Play-Doh, or Legos," I said, surprising myself with the number of different toys I could think of just off the top of my head—for someone who thinks she doesn't know anything about kids.

"Yeah," Nick said. This is the first time we've ever made a decision about a major purchase based on any information other than our own tastes and bankbook. Bit by bit, we are planning, making choices in shaping this environment to suit the person who's coming, whose own tastes (Matchbox cars? mudpies? a violin?) exist for the moment only in our imaginations.

♥

We're on the phone with Charles in San Francisco. Maybe, Nick says, the name "Charles Matthew"? "Do you know any good Virgo men?" I ask Charles. September 24, my due date, would be Libra, but I think the baby's going to be early.

"I don't know any good men," Charles says mildly after a pause. He hasn't had a relationship since he broke off with his previous partner four years ago.

"I mean," he resumes, "I'm sure there are some out there, like Nick Coles. But I don't know any. In general, it's a horrible species." He laughs. "You can't live with them, you can't shoot 'em."

꙳

Silence in the house this morning. Nine o'clock and the only sounds are birds — a very quiet morning. I'm relishing it.

I don't think Charlee gets much silence. But she gets other stuff. She gets the adoration of two little girls. She brought them by yesterday on their way to the zoo and Gillian was hanging on her. Ally is an elf, dancing her way through her life, always in search of new sensory pleasures. The three of them look like they have a lot of fun together.

I'm scaring myself again. Allowing myself to feel how good my life is.

Helen: "Were you letting yourself have too much fun? Is that why you feel depressed?"

I've been enjoying an uncharacteristic peace of mind in the past few months. I don't want it to be taken away from me. This fantasy of Job persists: even if I'm a really good girl, everything in my life might be taken away.

꙳

Went out yesterday and bought five dresses, all size L or XL, at a discount store. I can't believe the relief this purchase has given me. Now I don't have to worry what to wear at business meetings. Plus, none of them are those horrible pastel, ruffly "maternity" designs.

"All shall be well, and all shall be well, and all manner of thing shall be well." Julian of Norwich wrote that five hundred years ago, and it's still true. Von gave me a book of her writings for Christmas last year. I keep reading it over and over, but reading about faith is not the same as actually *having* faith. If only I could, from day to day, *have* faith that life will take care of itself, then I'd have peace of mind. It doesn't come naturally. It wasn't what I learned as a child. I learned to worry and obsess about everything that might go wrong. To focus on potential disasters rather than on the stuff happening right here and right now that might possibly be OK. I could worry and obsess about so many things right now: whether we'll have a renter for the third-floor apartment, whether the kid will be OK, whether we'll be able to buy the empty lot next door, how we'll manage moving to London for four months, and of course how to pay for it all. The endless anxiety about money, always independent of how much we actually have. Every time I look around the house I see more things to be done—cleaning, fixing. My office is in a perpetual state of clutter because I have so little shelving and storage space. Not a complaint, because I love doing things to and for the house, but a statement of a dilemma: How and when will I ever get everything done? Will we be able to pay for it all, with a baby on the way?

A hot day today, up to 90. The car is at the shop for a squeal in the right front wheel. I have a dentist's appointment at 1:15. Will I be able to cycle to the dentist, at six months pregnant, in 85-degree weather? I'm never sure of my physical capacities anymore.

Nick is so patient with me these days. Here we sit side by side in bed, writing. The mourning doves are calling softly outside the open window, and the humid sunny air promises a real summer day. We're poised on the threshold between spring and summer—it's evident in the mild twilights we've been having, and the sweet, cloying scent of the locust trees, which began to dangle their racemes of white pea-flowers five days or so ago. This moment in the season is always resonant to me, recalling some of the most carefree times of my life. Young times, when I didn't dwell on life's difficulties. The blissful ignorance of a delayed adolescence. The illusion is that peace is not a choice I make, but that it comes from nowhere—that it grows on trees, so to speak.

In fact, I see so much in my life that has occurred serendipitously, without my choosing. Business contracts I've secured, pieces I've written, story ideas that have dawned on me, people I've met, this kid I'm carrying. These pieces of life are like "volunteer" seedlings that just happen to pop up in the right space at the right time and grow to form the more valuable drifts of color and texture in the landscape.

The car, it turns out, is on its last leg. It didn't actually quit running, but what sounded like a little squeak in the right front wheel turned out to be a full set of front and rear brakes, an engine mount, a tie rod, a front-end alignment, and maybe another clutch. The car has only 56,000 miles. I was shocked at the $700 bill. Nick is convinced now we need to get a new car. An enormous, unexpected expense. It's at these moments that I'm tempted to ditch all the crap about "peace" and feel—however temporarily—as though the mooning I do in this journal is a lot of wasted (billable) time.

♆

Watched a two-hour movie on TV last night and Nick sat for the last forty-five minutes with his hand on my belly, feeling our baby kicking around. Often when I put Nick's hand on my belly the baby stops moving, as though he can tell Daddy's there and he calms down—though all the baby books say it's Mom who calms the baby down and Daddy who revs him up.

It's hard for Nick to feel our baby, though he was first able to feel him several weeks ago—we're now at week twenty-four. (Even now as I sit with the journal on my knee and it rests against my belly, the baby's kicks bounce it around.) Nick says—oh, a real thump!—Nick says he has to try to feel past my breathing, and the pulses in his own hand and in my belly. But the kid is getting so strong. And big. "Really a handful down there," Nick said at quarter to six this morning, as we lay like spoons in the early dawn. "Two handfuls, even." He just keeps growing and growing, and I have four more months to go! I sometimes worry about how much bigger he's going to get and whether my body can hold it. But I've handled it so far.

I felt so happy this morning to have a whole person who's part of Nick living inside of me. "Remember how disgusted I was in the beginning?" I said to him as I sniffed his chest, inhaling his musky scent. "I don't feel that way anymore." And he wondered at how pregnancy is a process that takes one through a range of feelings and physical states "in preparation for the rigors of living with a new being in one's life." I remember the time early on when I questioned whether I'd ever feel anything but truly disgusting—like a piece of tenderized meat.

For Nick, the process is more subtle. He says he can't get as clear a connection to our baby as I have because he can't feel or physically perceive the baby as clearly. "A big step was the ultrasound," he said. Now he can feel my belly, "which so obviously has something living in it," he said. But he said the other day that he's trying to get ready for the surge of feeling he knows will overtake him when the baby is born. "It will be like floodgates opening," he said. I try to imagine it.

He said it was a great relief to him to discover I was pregnant. I was surprised to hear this. He'd never mentioned this to me before. He said he had been ready. "I didn't know you were ready," I told him. We'd talked about it for more than two years and I'd never heard him articulate his readiness. He said he didn't know, either, until I took the test and it came out positive.

"I just felt so relieved," he said. "I felt we were finally getting on with it—like we were saying, *OK: let's go.*"

A quiet morning. Warm and damp after a constant overnight rain. I'm sure our rain barrel in the back garden is overflowing. The garden is very happy—peas flowering and producing fat pods, beans putting out new shoots each day, peppers blossoming, just waiting for bees to climb inside and drop some pollen. The sundrops are finally flowering, and the white foxgloves are nearing the end of their first blooming season. I started them eighteen months ago from seed! I'll let them go to seed and see what volunteers poke up. Summer solstice is in five days, but the gardens, in their voluptuousness, have arrived a few weeks early.

I went shopping downtown for Nick's Father's Day gift in my new sky-blue jersey dress. The bodice outlines my belly, and the scoopneck shows my new "cleavage." I drew stares from all kinds of people, and at times felt like a streetwalker—as though it were shameful for a pregnant woman to wear a dress that clings to her ripe figure. The pregnant woman's body is not an image people are used to seeing. Before pregnancy I saw images of myself everywhere—the slim young women on television, in ads, catalogs, and practically any print material, especially those trying to sell something through sex. I was "sexy." Now I'm nowhere. Every week, the image of my self is less and less apparent in the catalogs that come in the mail. I page through them with knowledge beforehand of the futility of turning their pages, but I look anyway, and I see nothing that will fit me, no image that tells me *You are here*, that confirms my location in the consumer world. I realize: how many women *always* feel this way, pregnant or not?—it's awful, the consumerist allure married with the sense of dislocation built into advertising. You're supposed to want all this beautiful stuff, the stuff will make you beautiful, yet you can't see anywhere a body that looks like your own. Pervasive, personal failure, page after page.

And I wonder, isn't the pregnant woman an untapped market?—4 million women each year. I guess the marketers stack that figure up against the general population, 250 million, and 4 million seems paltry. But I look through the pictures of bras and underwear and bathrobes and gowns in the Victoria's Secret catalog, which comes nearly every week (addressed to Nick), and wonder if they wouldn't boost sales even a bit by making some nice panties for pregnant women, some bathrobes and bathing suits and nighties that will fit over a pregnant belly, some halfway attractive nursing bras. Then I think about how Susan Faludi reported that men make up 30 to 40 percent of Victoria's Secret's walk-in clientele, and nearly half its sales volume, and I see one of the reasons that the pregnant body doesn't get a slot in their catalog: it's all about sex appeal from the traditional American masculine viewpoint. Imagine how it would change the tone of their catalog if they had pregnant women modeling a few outfits – not to speak of bras and bathing suits.

The dresses I bought are all size large. Except for the blue jersey one, which is extra-large. I bought them all on the sale rack at a discount store. My own snobbishness kills me: I'd never have thought of shopping there except that I needed clothes I could wear in hot weather; I needed them soon, so I didn't have time to make them; and I needed clothes that were cheap enough to buy "in bulk" (as it were). As I put my credit card on the counter I thought of my sister, who was already size large before she got pregnant, and who says she now has to go to "fat-lady stores" to get clothes that fit and that are reasonably priced. I felt sad that I could solve my problem so easily when there are so many other women who were at the mercy of high-priced maternity boutiques, or else Goodwill (at which I've bought two dresses and two pairs of shorts, for a total of less than ten dollars).

Aren't I still sexy? Nick thinks so, but I don't know about anyone else. Pregnant women's bellies are the most voluptuous sign of sex. How did

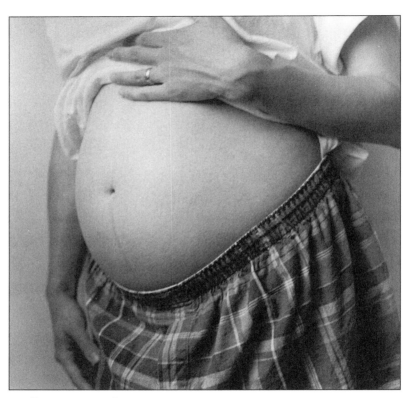

Twenty-six weeks pregnant.

I get this way, after all? And the full, round breasts. The culture divorces the functionality of breasts from their sexuality. We pregnant ladies are supposed to drape our bodies in floral print and lace, pleats that accentuate the belly's size but hide its contours. Babydoll clothes. "Seems like pregnancy is a world of pastels and fuzzy things," Nick said when we were just starting out. A pregnant woman thumbs her nose at social code when she claims her sexuality in any way publicly—when she wears a simple jersey dress that bares her collarbones and clings to her body. A dress that would pass unnoticed on a nonpregnant woman. This is why the *Vanity Fair* cover shot of Demi Moore naked and pregnant was so shocking—a naked, sexy pregnant woman! Or, rather, a sexy woman who happens to be pregnant. I've yet to see a pregnant woman on the street, in the store, on the bus, anywhere, who wasn't dressed in either one of two uniforms: black stretch-pants and big floral-print shirts, or else the blowsy gathered skirt attached to the empire waist, beruffled and belaced within an inch of her life.

I caught glimpses of myself in the shop windows: dark hair, dark eyes, legs still slim, belly round like a bowl, breasts full and firm for the first time in my life. I looked sexy, but in a different way than I used to. Less stringy, like a vine; more juicy and ripe, like the fruit.

My friend Sharon asked me if people were responding differently to me now that they can see that I'm pregnant. I said that women have been especially responsive and understanding, and that in places like an elevator or the grocery store they make room for me, give me understanding little smiles, make me feel part of a club or a team.

She talked about "showing." The four-letter word of pregnancy: "show." Such a loaded little word, with connotations of voyeurism and exhibitionism—come on, give us a little peek, show us what you've got. "You hardly show at all," people are always telling me. It makes me feel as though a million unseen eyes are on me, waiting for me to "do" something. Sharon says she went to a beach when she was seven months pregnant with Brian, her only child, who's now seventeen. "I had a maternity bathing suit on and everything," she said, "and people still told me I had no business 'parading' and 'showing' my body in public. I wasn't supposed to 'show' so much.

"But I was in rock bands almost up until the time I had Brian," she said. When she began to "show," her friends started making sure she got the most comfortable seat. As though she'd suddenly become weak, she said. But she enjoyed the times people made room for her on buses.

"I played my guitar," she said, "until I could no longer reach around my belly."

♥

Just read an essay about doing nothing: waiting, leisure. The author calls pregnancy "the great while."

I really am waiting. While each day passes, as our baby gets bigger and stronger and kicks me harder, making himself and his will known to me in these initial strugglings, I almost palpably feel my life and self being changed, molded, into something I can't control or even comprehend: motherhood. A mother, a person whose consciousness is fully attuned to the care of another person. A person whose own well-being is intertwined with another's. I have the sense of needing to sit still while this change comes over me, the way the world quiets down before a storm blows through, the silence before the earthquake or volcanic eruption. For a while, the storm or the eruption hurts and upsets everything. In the long run, though, it makes the entire environment richer.

Nick followed me down to the back porch with his journal this morning. Often, lately, he doesn't want to be apart from me. I considered going back into the house to meditate. But soon I'll have another person with me all the time, on the outside, clamoring for my attention. No matter how the saying goes about praying alone in a closet, from now on I'd better learn to do everything I need to do for my own well-being in the company of at least one other person.

One worry still nags at me, though: that Nick and I will never make love again. That we'll never be alone again.

The stronger this kid gets, the more afraid of him I become. It's complicated, though—I don't want him to be weak; I *want* him to be strong. When he belts me (as he's been doing this past week) I feel glad that he has spirit, a strong physical constitution, and apparently a good deal of persistence. It's simultaneously frightening, not least because it's a boy—and he's kicking me from the inside out, increasingly packing a wallop. "Does it hurt?" Nick asked today, and before he asked it this had never occurred to me. Maybe it'll actually begin to hurt. Right now, it's just uncomfortable, but the books say pregnancy can get painful in the last trimester. Twenty-six weeks—I'll be there in two more days. And when this little man begins to hurt me there will be nothing I can do but sit back and take it. Something I'm not used to doing anymore with men (little or big).

And if he's making this much fuss before he's born, what might he do afterward?

Von says Carter was very active before he was born and turned out to be a "good" baby, an "easy" baby, which really means a quiet baby. Maybe it's because I don't know babies, but mine seems so wild already that I sometimes have visions of epilepsy, seizures, or just a temperament never satisfied. My dream is to put him in a "baby sling" on the front of me, walk around London, visit the museums, sit down for tea, feed him, and read and write in my journal. Take him on long walks. Be able to talk to him and sing to him and not cause him to cry. Who knows whether his temperament will allow us to spend days like this? Kathryn Rhett talks about how the trauma of her daughter's birth made it impossible for them to take a walk and have a visitor both in the same day, even when her daughter was months old. Her daughter would lie awake screaming with overstimulation and what Brazelton calls "disorganization" the entire night. She couldn't even gaze for too long at the mobile hanging over her crib or she'd lose it.

Our lives, our peace destroyed. *My* peace. Because I'm the flexible one, the one who works at home, I will be the one who will have to deal with any problem or disorder. My environment shattered. I've come to cherish silence and the inward life that comes from long hours alone with words, and the deep stillness of Quaker Meeting. It would be just my luck to get a kid who would dismantle all the structures I've built to help me.

Here I go again, worrying about everything that can go *wrong*. What mother does best.

I woke up this morning feeling like somebody had taken a crowbar to my neck and shoulders, yet the silence of our house restores me and makes me happy. The silence is my organizing principle. It's not absolute silence — within it are the trees' leaves rustling in the air, warm and fragrant now with hawthorn and honeysuckle; the cut grass rasping under my rubber flip-flops as I pad across the lot next door to check on my bean plants, basil, and peppers; the birds singing to each other in a Sunday morning chorus. The familiar, almost ritualistic sounds of tea making: the rattle of the kettle lid coming off, the rush of water rinsing out the pot, the scrape of butterknife against bread. These are the sounds that organize my brain. I'm not sure what I'll do if my baby can't bear the sights and sounds of my life. Or if he just screams all the time and takes away the silence. I know I'll feel compelled to give up my life. That's what I think of when I think of "mother": a person who organizes everything in her life around her family, with such little time to herself. A person who gives up everything for other people, and who is so unhappy about it.

Third Trimester

Twenty-six weeks along, today. Exactly three and a half months till due date.

Dreamed last night that Nick and I came home and found the house burglarized. The living room windows had been forced open. But nothing had been stolen — just our privacy invaded.

✋

I didn't realize how much more physically vulnerable I feel now that I'm heavily pregnant, until this colleague of Nick's from Louisiana came two days ago to stay for a week. Another of

Nick's colleagues was supposed to put him up, but he can only do it for the guy's second week here. And Nick's teaching out of town and spending weeknights forty-five miles away, so it's just me and the guy in the house. It's totally weird to have another man in the house without having Nick. The guy's a martial arts expert and very masculine, not exactly macho but pretty physically powerful, and it feels bizarre having him in the house while Nick is away. Not that there's been any direct threat. He's nice and just goes about his business, though he spent last evening hanging around in the kitchen, and I just wanted some dinner and some peace and quiet after a very long, hot day.

I mean, I guess being from Louisiana, 95 degrees is nothing to him, but to me it's too fucking hot even to think, much less attempt to be a scintillating conversationalist. It's so hot and humid that I'm having a lot of trouble working. I got nothing accomplished this morning but a few household chores, some hand wash, and my glucose-tolerance meal for my gestational diabetes blood test at the birth center. The midwives' handbook says $1\frac{1}{2}$ percent of pregnant women get diabetes while they're pregnant, and this means every woman has to get blood drawn for a screening at the end of roughly twenty-four weeks — six months. I wasn't allowed to eat anything before 10:30, and then at exactly 10:30 I had to eat two scrambled eggs, two slices of toast, a cup of milk, and half a cup of orange juice, and nothing else. It was so hot and I was so starved from not being allowed to eat *anything* for four hours after waking that I was practically blacking out over the gas burner, spatula in hand. My hands were shaking as I gulped the eggs down. I could have eaten a whole dozen. If I hadn't had to be home to eat on time I would have gone somewhere air-conditioned to read or write (and, of course, eat, and eat, and eat).

☙

Went for the six-month checkup today and had Kathy McKain again. I asked her for some better pregnancy reading than *Expecting the Worst.* It's comprehensive, for sure, but it's driving me crazy with its lists of everything that can go wrong. I'm too obsessive to read it.

"I know a lot of people like those prescriptive books," Kathy said, almost apologetically, "but I still use *Spiritual Midwifery.* It has a lot of old hippie language, which some people don't feel comfortable with, but I'm old enough to have used that kind of language myself, and I like it. It's the only book I've found that has pictures of actual women, and the women tell their stories in their own words." Just what I was looking for to begin with. I wondered if Nan, hippie that she was, read this book when she was having Sam and Simon. Kathy lends her copy out to pregnant women at the center because, she says, "There's nothing like a *story* to tell you what to expect, and how it feels to go through this process."

Nick and I usually go together to all our checkups. This time, since he's away teaching, I went by myself, and it was nice for a change to speak with the midwife alone, just us two women in the room. I told Kathy I'm worried because the baby sometimes moves so hard and rough, that sometimes I have ugly ideas that he has epilepsy because my whole belly shakes and then suddenly stops. No baby I've ever seen does stuff like that. Plus, I thought I wasn't supposed to see it on the outside until I was about eight months pregnant.

"Is it normal?" I asked. "I don't think I've asked that question so many times in my life before I got pregnant."

She said the baby moves in coordinated ways that establish neurological pathways throughout his body, and that the stronger the movements are, the better. She used the Doppler to listen to the heartbeat again. It was 144 beats per minute today. She taught me the difference between the beating of the umbilical cord and the sound of the baby's heart itself. The cord produces the *whoosh-whoosh* sound we've been hearing for months. The heart produces a sharper knocking, and we heard that clearly today. She measured my uterus from pelvic bone to "fundus"—the top of the uterus, where Kathy said the placenta is usually attached—and it was twenty-seven centimeters, or about ten and a half inches. Amazing how it grows!

"You don't look like you stick out that much," Jeri said later when I told her my uterus was almost a foot high.

"It's not sticking out—it's sticking up against my lungs."

I asked Kathy to show me how much bigger my belly would get. She arched her hand to a point about four inches from my belly. "I better get bigger dresses," I said. She pulled the dress out a bit at the waist and said, "Oh, I don't think you'll need bigger dresses."

Kathy massaged my belly, trying to determine the baby's position. I'd read that he's supposed to settle into a head-down position soon. Most of the books urge you not to worry if your baby hasn't shifted into the "vertex" position by the seventh month—"There's plenty of time for the baby to shift positions or be rotated manually," the sort of line designed to comfort that ends up doing just the opposite: you read it and get the feeling that there really *isn't* that much time after all. Nobody wants a breech birth or, worse, a lateral presentation, when the hand or shoulder wants to come out first. Kathy dug her fingers between my hipbones and asked me to take a large breath and let it out. As I exhaled she sank her fingertips gently into the space around the cervix, and felt around. She felt the back of the head facing front-wards, and a bit to the right, with his body curled around to the right and the legs coming down on the left. I tried to feel the head myself but couldn't. She said that feeling my own belly flexed my abdominal muscles, and this prevented me from feeling his head.

Then Kathy moved the Doppler stick to the top of my belly and got a cavernous sound, like the inside of a seashell.

"You hear the storm?" she said.

It did sound like a storm, wind and rain whipping through a tangle of trees and brush.

"That's the placenta," she said. "It's full of blood, and it sounds like a storm."

Just back from a team meeting at Jeri's. At the door she couldn't help but touch my belly again. I think these dresses make a difference. They're pretty, and they show my belly more than Nick's jeans ever did. Today I wore the floral cotton one with the crinkly skirt. The weather is almost unbearably hot, and this dress is the coolest one I bought. I like the big, comfortable clothes I've been discovering. In a way, being pregnant has introduced me to a new world of clothes. For three or four months, I haven't worn anything with a waistband, except for

Nick's big jeans. I've forgotten what it feels like to be bound up like that. I actually might not want to go back.

✋

Luisa called today to schedule our next walk. She said her forehead is still growing a big mole despite a laser surgery scheduled for last week. "It was too intense for the laser," she said.

"Too intense?" I asked.

"It was *too big,*" she said bluntly. "It's out of control. I have to have it removed next week," by which I suppose she meant cut off. Hadn't the dental hygienist said, of the so-called pregnancy tumors, "They don't go away—you have to have them *cut* off"?

"Gosh," I said, "how awful." By way of commiserating I told her the rash was still on my legs, and that I was unbearably hot and unable to sleep.

"And does your skin itch?" she asked. "I mean, not from the rash, but just by itself, from the skin stretching?"

"Yeah, my belly itches all the time now."

"God: we are *falling apart,* Jen," she said. "Just falling apart. But we'll get through it. Millions of women have."

"I know," I said, "I keep having to remind myself that women have done this for millennia. Not just for centuries, but *millennia.*"

After lunch Janey called. We don't really travel in the same circles and haven't run into each other for four months. Back then I was still in a panic of disgust and confusion. "I'm just calling to check up on you," she said. I told her frankly that pregnancy has been the greatest thing to happen to me. That it has made me hopeful.

"It's making me an optimist," I said.

"Didn't I tell you?" she said enthusiastically. "Wait till he's born. It only gets better. I want to see this little boy—after all, I'm the first person besides Nick who knew about him."

Then Charlee came over for our sixteenth photo shoot. It's hard to believe we've been doing this for four months. I was wearing the bright green plaid boxer shorts I bought for a dollar at the Goodwill, and a big T-shirt. She had me tuck the shirt in so she could capture the garish plaid, what she called "the golf esprit" of the shorts. I pulled the waistband below my belly. Charlee laughed. "If I didn't have the knowledge of the rest of your body and you didn't have boobs," she said, "you would look just like a fifty-year-old guy with a beer gut in this shot." It was a great session. We talk more and more about our lives.

When I was a daily journalist, I was taught to keep my distance from the people I wrote about. Working with Charlee has taught me the necessity, and the common sense, of breaking down that pretense of objectivity—because it doesn't exist anyway; of building relationships with the people whose stories you're telling. I've watched her put it into practice with me. Her friendship and our work together have given me a way to make sense of my unexpected pregnancy, and to grow affectionate toward an unseen being about whom I'd initially felt such fear, disgust, and resentment.

✋

Talked to Judy today. In her sixth month now, she's feeling better physically, except for a lot of water retention. "My ankles are gone," she said.

"I looked down at my legs the other day, and I thought, 'Something's different here.' Then I noticed that from my thighs down to my feet was a straight line. I don't have any ankles anymore." Her feet are so swollen that it hurts her even to wear tennis shoes.

Last week she came down with a head cold. She called Tim at work to ask him what she could take for a stuffy nose and headache. "He's like, 'Did you see my handout?' He has all these lists of helpful hints for pregnant women. He types up—what are they called?—'protocols' for the nurses to hand out for different problems."

"So did he tell you what you could take?"

"I told him I didn't have any handout. He's like, 'It's on the computer at home.' I was like, 'Can't you just *tell* me?' But he couldn't remember the exact stuff. So I went on the computer and found the list. You can take Sudafed, and only Sudafed—not the stuff with ibuprofen or anything else in it—and Afrin nasal spray, and that's, like, it."

I got addicted to Afrin once. Afrin made it easier to breathe for about five minutes, and after that I felt like somebody had sealed my nose with duct tape, and I realized I was going to need twice as much Afrin every five minutes for the rest of my life ever to breathe again. Forget Sudafed, too—it just makes me feel like I'm breathing helium.

Judy says the physical curveballs pregnancy has thrown her have made Tim better able to empathize with his patients. "He can tell them, week by week, 'This is when you'll start to feel like this, and this is when you'll start to feel like that. I know, because my wife is pregnant.' " Judy says the patients love it, and so do the nurses. The doctors are amazed that their new colleague is planning to attend child-birth classes with his pregnant wife.

"All the doctors were laughing at him," she said. "My doctor was incredulous when I told him Tim was coming to the classes with me. He was like, 'I can't believe that, I'd never go to those things.' I told him I wasn't making Tim do it. I gave Tim the choice, and he said he wanted to do it."

"What did the doctor say when you told him that?"

"He was like, 'I'm going to have a talk with him. He shouldn't have to do that.' But the nurses were all like, 'Oh—Tim's *great!* He's going to childbirth classes with his wife, isn't that wonderful?' "

I thought of my and Nick's first childbirth class this week, all the charts about labor stages, and drawings of a pregnant woman's innards, squashed together and color-keyed—yellow for the bladder, red for the uterus, gray for the lungs. Why are the drawings in books and on posters always headless and legless, as though the rest of the pregnant woman's body never matters? Our instructor, Sylvia, demonstrated the cervix's dilation to ten centimeters by using a coffee can encased in a tube sock: as she slowly pulled the sock off the can, the elastic around the narrow sock top widened and finally stretched to the perimeter, leaving us looking into an empty Maxwell House can. "That's ten cen-timeters, by the way," Sylvia said with a sly smile, and three of the four women in the room who had not yet had any children shifted in our seats, as though our crotches were already stinging. The fourth woman just grinned. Sylvia warned us not to push if the cervix is not fully dilated. It's not only painful, she said, but it also actually prolongs your labor because it bruises and swells the cervix, shrinking its opening—preventing that last little bit of dilation. Even nine and a half centimeters is not full dilation, Sylvia said. How much could half a centimeter matter?—it's like a quarter of an inch, for God's sake, isn't it? I was not the only one who groaned, and suddenly I had the urge to pee. "I think I have to go to the bathroom now," I said, and the room erupted in laughter as I stood, but I was looking at the can and wondering how the little tiny cervix would open that wide without causing me utter agony. When they taught me how to insert a diaphragm, they told me to check for my covered cervix by probing for a knob that feels like the tip of my nose. How could the tip of my nose stretch to the width of a coffee can? Maybe a forty-eight-hour migraine was better, after all. "That's really hard," I mumbled, casting one last look at the can and heading for the bathroom.

I guess there's no new fact that childbirth class could teach Tim about female anatomy, but it might, if nothing else, be a relaxing two hours in each other's company. I had watched the other guys affectionately massaging their wives' backs during the class; one guy in particular, a young man about twenty-four or so, couldn't keep his arm from stealing around his wife's shoulders, and she leaned against him in fatigue and closed her eyes.

"I wonder how Tim will feel when he gets in there, and you're having the baby, and he's out of control?" I asked. "I mean, he's not going to deliver the baby. He's going to be out of control."

"He doesn't *want* to be in control," Judy said. "But he'll be way more freaked out than I am, I'm sure. He's more hyper than I ever expected him to get." A few weeks ago, she said, she got called to sub for her old volleyball team. She hadn't played volleyball for months. "So I *played,*" she said, and I could hear the relief in her voice. Just like hearing the tinge of envy in Luisa's voice at lunch today when she asked a friend of ours how much she'd been running lately.

"How did it feel?" I asked Judy.

"It was *great,*" she said. "I played for two hours." Worked up the sweat she used to on a weekly basis. "I didn't tell Tim for a week, then I just happened to mention it. And he went *off* on me: 'How could you do this, somebody could have knocked you down, you could have fallen, something terrible could have happened,' blah blah blah. I was like, 'What's going on, you let me mow the grass, you let me scrape the ceiling and paint it, why can't I play volleyball?'" I was struck by the word *let.* It's a word that shows up a lot in the chapters to the Expectant Father in Dr. Bradley's old-fashioned pregnancy book—something like, "Don't *let* her iron all your shirts at once; tell her to iron two or three and then take a rest." Nick had read that and said, to the hypothetical Future Father, "Why the hell don't you iron your own shirts?"

"And I was like, 'Besides, everybody was staying away from me, believe me, nobody was going to touch me, *everybody* on the court knew I was pregnant.'"

"When he starts acting like a doctor with me, I just get really upset with him. He's not supposed to do that. It's not part of his job. He's not supposed to treat family or friends."

I wonder how Tim can *not* act like a doctor. Tim has a true calling to obstetrics and gynecology and years of technical study and clinical experience. How's he supposed to distance himself from his own wife's and kid's situation? The ultrasound, for instance, showed that their baby has an irregular heartbeat. Tim isn't in Nick's position. He can't just hold Judy's hand and stare starstruck at the screen in blissful ignorance. He can't watch the wiggling form and feel blown away by the introduction, as though he's meeting his kid for the first time. He's probably looked at hundreds of sonograms. He's trained to recognize immediately the brain, the heart, the spine, bone density, cranial and thoracic circumferences, all the attributes the midwives' OB pointed out for us on our sonogram. His training makes him measure everything he sees by all the gestational-age statistics he knows. Except in this case his training just pours gasoline on the spark lit by his feelings.

"He got real quiet during the ultrasound, and I knew something was wrong," Judy said. "Then later on the neonate who lives two doors down from us told us probably the heart just was immature, it hadn't formed completely yet, that he sees this kind of thing all the time and it turns out fine," which Tim most likely already knows, and has even told other patients. But this time his wife is the patient and the fetus with the potential problem is his own kid.

"After we left the doctor's office, Tim wouldn't say a word. Then we went to dinner, and I said, 'Tell me what's wrong. Tell me what you're thinking.' And he went through all this stuff about the ultrasound and the heartbeat. And then he said, 'But the brain looks really good — it's a *really good brain.*' And I was like, 'I didn't know you were worrying about the brain or the heart, or whatever.' And he was like, 'Well, I don't know how much you want to know,' and I was like, 'I want to know whatever you know! Don't just sit there and not tell me!' " So they talked about it.

Knowledge is power, but it is also innocence lost. Tim has seen all kinds of things go wrong, which is why he was reluctant to tell his family and friends until the beginning of her second trimester that Judy was pregnant. The average 25 percent chance of miscarriage in the first thirteen weeks was just too high for his comfort. I congratulated him, and he said, a line appearing on his usually smooth forehead, "For what?"

"We'll be in there," Judy predicts of her labor, "and every time a monitor goes off or something, he's going to know what it means, and I won't have a clue."

I told her I couldn't wait to meet my niece. I told her I expected she would be beautiful. "Look at the two of you— " I began, but she cut me off. "I can't think about this now, I think I have to go," she said. I asked her why she was so abrupt.

"I just am not behaving in the way I always thought I would grow up to be," she said. "I thought I would get all mushy when I was going to have a baby. But I'm, like, so detached."

"But you're not a mushy kind of person. You're pragmatic," I said. "You're not a romantic."

"I used to be a romantic. But I'm not anymore."

"But you'll get attached once she comes along."

"I know I will, but until that happens, I just don't want to think about it," she said, nettled.

"Let yourself fall in love with her a little bit, Jude," I said. "She's coming. She's already here."

"No, she's not," she protested, "not yet."

They have a name for her. They're not telling anyone what it is. "We haven't actually talked about whether we're telling anyone or not," she said. "But we've only told people who live far away."

I told her we don't have a name yet. "You *don't?*" she said.

"No. We've been poring over a baby name book, making lists, but nothing sounds right. We have a bunch that we're thinking about, but I think we'll have to meet him first. I think we'll have to see his face before we call him anything."

She snorted with laughter. "Well, I have something to tell you, Jenny," she said. Nobody calls me Jenny anymore—my childhood name. "He's not going to look like very much when he comes out. He's not going to look *anything* like what he'll end up looking like. So why do you need to see his *face?*"

I broke down today and actually went to one of those maternity shops. I bought a bathing suit. The one I bought was the only one I considered buying—a simple black-and-purple suit with a V-neck. All the others had strange gathered panels around the belly, or silly little skirts, or were made of bad polka-dotted fabric or floral prints. This one is plain. It looks like a suit a nonpregnant woman might wear, except for the leg holes, which are low and make my legs look short.

I dragged Nick into the fitting room to help me decide whether to buy a small or medium. All the books say you're supposed to buy stuff in your "pre-pregnancy size," which would be medium, but the medium is so loose in the bust. The sales woman told me to buy the medium because my belly will need the room to grow into by September, but she didn't like the idea of my breasts not getting "support." They are, after all, size B now. Size B! — and they may get even bigger yet. I tried on the small — it fit in the bust but it left no room for my belly to grow. "It's going to be too small soon. You're going to gain another five pounds," Nick said.

I put the medium back on.

"It's so baggy in the bum," he said. "Your bum's not going to get any bigger."

I pulled at the leg holes, tugging them up a bit in a French-cut line, and said, "For fifty bucks, the leg cut is so disappointing."

"Yeah," he said, "it's as though whoever makes these things doesn't think you'll want to look the least bit sexy." Or doesn't think I *could*, even if I wanted to.

As I looked at myself in the three-way mirror, though, I was pretty proud of myself. I've gained fifteen pounds, and I think I'll put on more than five in this last trimester. All the books say you should gain a pound a week in the last two months. I think I'll get my old body back. At the same time, I don't feel fixated on being "small" or "thin" the way I used to. I realize I'm proud of myself not because I might be "thin" again, but because I'll get back to the body I used to feel so at home in. Doubtless there will be changes to that body — bigger hips and waist, I'll bet, and something has to change with these breasts that are now so big; can they really just shrivel back up again? — but I'll be prepared to accept these changes as results of this process. How can your body not change irrevocably as a result of somebody *living inside it* for nine months?

While we were in the maternity shop I noticed a young woman about twenty-six or twenty-seven trying on dresses. A very small woman, about five feet three, normally a size 4 or so, with short, thick brown hair and gorgeous brown eyes. She was carrying a powder-blue leather Coach purse and wearing lots of gold jewelry. Her husband was with her, helping her decide on a dress. After some back-and-forth between the fitting room and the rack, and a less-than-satisfying walk in front of the three-way mirror, she settled on an orange floral-print dress with an empire waist and skirt above the knee, but she hardly seemed keen on it. "Now, I want to explain the exchange policy to you," the saleswoman said, "because it's very strict." No cash refunds, only in-store credit, the sole exception being charge-card purchases, which could be credited to the account. No exchanges after ten days. Ten days! Whatever happened to that good old American maxim, "The customer is always right"? When you're pregnant, it's "Caveat emptor." The maternity shop is the only store where the customer's always wrong. The cashier made the woman sign the policy printed on the back of the receipt.

Judy told me she went through this at a maternity shop in Cleveland. When she protested that she was only four months pregnant and didn't know whether the dress she'd just bought for a wedding would fit in a month, she said the clerk told her, "Get used to it, honey — this is the way *all* maternity stores are."

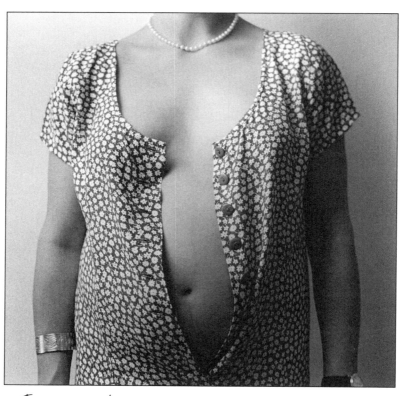

Twenty-six weeks pregnant.

Went for my Rhogam shot today. The nurses call it The Shot and say it will keep my Rh-negative blood from making antibodies that will kill the baby's blood, in case he has Rh-positive blood like Nick's. I have to get The Shot again after he's born, if his blood is positive, in case I want to have another kid and don't want to have my blood reject it as a foreign body and trigger a spontaneous abortion—a "miscarriage."

Later, a woman wearing a blue hospital gown over regular clothes nearly walked into me on her way out of the elevator. "Jeez!" she said, sidestepping, "it seems like *everybody* I see these days is pregnant. I hope that don't mean nothin'," she added, "I don't want to be havin' no more babies."

"I don't think it means anything," I said.

"Well, honey, you carry it real well."

"Can we fit one more in here?" I asked the pack in the elevator, hoping to squeeze in after my appointment. A tall guy stepped back a bit to make room while the woman beside him said, her eyebrows rising significantly, "Looks like one-and-a-half more."

I was wearing the little one-piece rayon floral-print minidress I'd bought at the Goodwill for two dollars. It has a low scoopneck and very short sleeves, the rayon drapes close to my breasts and belly, and the short skirt falls mid-thigh. Having worn only long skirts for the past three weeks and Nick's jeans before that, this dress keeps me really cool, but I also feel a little bit naked in it, which is weird because I wouldn't feel that way if I weren't pregnant. As I walked out of the hospital, every single man stared at me—the custodians, the visitors, the patients, the shuttle driver sitting in his bus parked at the front door. I was thankful for my sunglasses, so I didn't have to meet anyone's eyes. Does nobody know what a pregnant woman's body looks like? But the stares were not disapproving. It was good to feel my body being appreciated again, and I was left with the conviction that another function of maternity clothes is to desexualize us. "You could wear that again *after*," the nurse said. Maternity clothes, everyone agrees, you throw away.

Been lazy this weekend. The baby is getting bigger all the time, so I get tired around midday and have to nap around 3 or 4. With the recent hot weather, I have a feeling these days of being in high summer in my body. The heart carrying its peak load; my body warmer even than Nick's—he had to wrap up in a blanket and pajamas in bed last night, while I wore a T-shirt and nothing else. Feeling like a poppy that has shed its petals to uncover a swelling seed capsule.

We saw a Czech film called *Kolya* last evening. The little boy's face was amazing. In watching the relationship between the boy and the musician, I was able to visualize concretely for the first time how deeply I might come to love our little guy.

It's Friday morning and I should be at my computer, working. Or else I should be cleaning my study or the house. But instead I'm sitting in the all-women-owned coffeehouse in Shadyside eating spinach-ricotta pie and writing for the first time this week.

I like this place because the food is good and you get free refills on the iced tea, because they have a clapped-out old couch that's easy on my back, because it's nonsmoking, and because it's never loud. I know the woman behind the counter. Nick is on her dissertation committee. ("Nick is such a sweetheart," she confides, in her Brooklyn accent. "He never asks me how the diss is coming. Just says hello.") When Von and I discovered it on one of our bike rides, she was so delighted with it that she inquired about buying a share in the collective. And one of the first things Von noticed: "There's a high chair in the corner. We can bring our baby here."

I'd like to take a kick at the baby. Kick him out. This morning I thought he was going to bruise my bladder or cause some other internal injury. He was doing karate kicks or chops or something. Nick watched him from the outside and was pretty surprised. I've gotten over whatever awe I used to feel and now feel impatience. Especially at the hiccups— can't stand the rhythmic twitching in my belly. It's like a faucet dripping while you're trying to sleep. Twitch . . . twitch . . . twitch. God! "Leave me alone!" I yelled this morning, and he actually stopped for a couple of minutes. And of course I felt guilty. "I yelled at him," I said to Nick. Probably the first of millions of times I'll yell at him in the next eighteen years. I get afraid it's a voice that's ingrained in me, that mother-voice: The Yell.

But I remember Helen's words: "You will yell, but you'll be able to say you're sorry for it. Being able to apologize means everything."

My mother came over Monday afternoon after her checkup at the oncologist's, with Dad. I had invited them to stop by. Her doctor's office is six blocks from our house, yet in two-and-a-half years of check-ups she hasn't stopped by once. I've been wondering all this time why she doesn't drop by, even just for twenty minutes, when she has an appointment six blocks from our house. I don't feel like I can ask her why. These cancer checkups make her so nervous that even alluding to them upsets her, and no one talks about them. I asked her how she was coming along at a picnic at Joe's the other day, and her jaw tightened.

I made tea. Mom says the doctor doesn't want to see her for another six months — she's doing so well in her recovery. She looks healthy and strong, but, as always, she didn't say much else about her doctor's visit. I had questions, but I didn't ask.

She didn't ask about our baby. She never asked me how I was, how I was feeling, how the baby is doing. On the other hand, she told me all about Judy's baby. "Every time I call Judy," she told me, "I ask how the baby is, and Judy says she kicks like mad."

Why didn't she ask about my baby?

I feel so angry when I think about it.

It doesn't matter; I can tell myself all kinds of rational explanations (she was, after all, coming from a checkup with her oncologist, enough to scare the shit out of anybody), but they don't matter — I can't help but feel hurt that she didn't ask about our baby, and take it personally, like it was my fault.

I must have done or said something to upset her. That's just the way it is between us — I can be so outspoken and tactless, and I say or do something that upsets her; then she gets overwhelmed by hurt feelings, and tells other people but shuts up around me. And then there's this Grand Canyon in our communication. I'll probably hear about it from Judy or Dad.

✵

I'm sitting naked in bed at 11:30 at night. It's still above 80 outside. In the 90-degree heat, my legs cramped three times today.

I have the air conditioner on in my study and a fan blowing right on me. I never used to sit in bed naked because I'd be so conscious of (and embarrassed by) any bulge in my belly, and I'd put on at least a shirt. I hope I never feel that kind of discomfort or shame about my body again. I wonder whether it will come back; whether being pregnant has once and for all given me a way to accept my body.

My breasts are three times their normal size. My belly is so big that, when I'm standing up, I have to crane my neck to see my feet. I've gained seventeen pounds—the same amount that Mom gained when she had Judy. She gained fifteen with me, sixteen with Joe. If I were going to be just like Mom, I wouldn't gain an ounce from here on out. But I have more than two months to go! Mom always said her pregnancies actually made her *thinner*. "It's the best diet," she always told me, "because there's a definite *end* to it. I lost weight with each one of you. I always ended up being thinner than I started out." How thoroughly she'd internalized the cultural pressure to be "thin"—and how eagerly I had always accepted that value when she passed it along to me. I've done so much hard work these past years to limit the compulsion to objectify my own body and begin to enjoy living in my own skin. It's so deeply ingrained, though, that I sometimes think I will be working against that compulsion for the rest of my life—always seeing my body as others might see it, rather than experiencing it from my own viewpoint.

I was right. Dad says that Mom was upset that I'd asked about her health that day at Joe's. I'd asked when her next appointment was. I'd asked how she was feeling. Dad says she doesn't like to talk about her health. Part of her recovery these past three years, he says, lies in not having to talk about cancer, or talking about it on her own terms. Sometimes, I spend months not knowing how she is. "How's your mother?" people ask, and I don't really know, but I always say she seems OK. "Don't I have a right to know how she is?" I asked Dad, then immediately felt ashamed. He said, gently but with some iron in his voice, "I don't know about rights, Jen, OK? All I know is, she needs not to talk about it." He told me if, in the future, I wanted to know anything, I could ask him. I asked him to tell her I'm sorry. I wish I could tell her myself. It grieves me that I hurt her so unwittingly.

Yet it also bugs me that we can't talk about it. She can't say, "I just don't want to talk about this, Jen." This is what I would want to do with my own kid. Maybe she's ashamed that she doesn't want to talk about it; maybe she's afraid of hurting me; maybe she doesn't know what she feels clearly enough to talk about it. I bet she's afraid of making me angry. I'd like to bring it up with her, but now I don't want to make her discuss her illness, or even think about it if she doesn't want to — this certainly should be her prerogative.

I don't know whether my mother and I will ever be able to talk about things that are important to us with frankness and without fear of hurting or being hurt.

This all just makes my head hurt worse. Yet I don't feel sick.

What is it I just read this morning that Kirkegaard said? — "Pregnancy is a time of paradox." Two persons in one. Pain and peace. I have a migraine; yet here I sit, like a Buddha, naked on my bed, my belly and breasts hanging: content.

He moves around inside me, shoves a foot into my ribs, elbows my bladder, making it sting.

I want to see his face.

☙

Unable to get my thoughts together for the past few weeks. Almost in my eighth month; in general, feeling content and even-tempered. Uncomfortable when the heat and humidity are high. He's getting very big now and kicks my ribs, my bladder. I almost peed by accident the other day. But I can't complain. I'm having an easy time of it.

Some days, or even moments during the day, though, I don't know what's happening to me. I'll have spent eight hours working, and I will try to eat in the heat by myself, because Nick's still away teaching, and suddenly I'll be overwhelmed by the fear of his not surviving the drive home and I'll want to call him to see if he's still alive. He has seventeen years on me, and I think more than ever these days about how he could die so far ahead of me. I stood in the kitchen and cried about this on Wednesday night. Ten o'clock at night and I had to fight the compulsion to call his B&B and wake him, just to make sure he was still around. Sometimes, I hound him to take care of himself so that he will still be around. Premonitions of our kid losing his father, the way Dad lost his when he was just seven years old.

I try to relax and talk back to these voices but I can rarely collect my thoughts. My mind seems too fluid to be collected, even by language. It's not just the fatigue and backache, the leg cramps and lack of sleep, though that's part of it. My mind's eye simply seems to be trained inward.

We've had a large rain. The tomatoes are growing fat on their vines, the fat fruit slumping the plants' spines — like mine. I shake off the rain and stake them, tying them gently with soft cotton strips to avoid chafing the stems' skin with twine.

"What is happening to me?" I sometimes think. I say this aloud sometimes, standing in the kitchen or in the garden, or trying to organize my weeks on my calendar. Not so many left now until he comes — six, seven, eight. Maybe more, but I don't think he will be late. (I persist in thinking he will be early, though everybody tells me first babies are late.) I forget to record my billable hours, or else I just *don't.* The book seems too difficult to open or to find in my study or my bag. I record them every other day, every three days, in batches, and I know they're accurate, but I still feel ashamed. I used to behave so scrupulously.

"What is happening to me?"

Fingertips ruffling the hairline at the back of my neck, wondering. I can't get it together.

I buy carriers for him. I've got all these carriers: an infant car-seat for up to twenty-two pounds, a big-boy car-seat for up to forty-eight pounds (how old will he be when he tips the scales at forty-eight?), an aluminum backpack. I price baby slings at Babyland. I keep my eyes peeled for interesting strollers: I want the one in which he can sleep, and into which I can pack my stuff. Do I have crib sheets? — do we have the room set up? — do I have a playpen? — no. We are going to *move,* this kid and I. We're not going to sit around. He's going to see his world.

I know this desire to take our baby places comes from having seen so little of the world as a child myself. Because I didn't go to kindergarten, and because we had no neighbors, I didn't even know any kids besides Joe and Judy until I was nearly six. It also comes from Mom telling me so many times how isolated she felt when we were small. How much she loved us, but how despairing she was at times that there were only baby voices to talk to. "I felt like I was going crazy, singing 'Twinkle, Twinkle, Little Star' all day. Your father would come home from work, and I'd make him sit at the kitchen table and talk to me," she'd tell me. "He'd say, 'What do you want to talk about?' *'Anything,'* I'd tell him. 'Just say *anything.* It doesn't have to *mean* anything. Just give me an adult voice to listen to.' " Ten hours a day, alone in the house. Can I manage to be a parent without that level of frustration? Is it right for me to put him into child care so that I can have a break? Each day, I promise myself that I will not let that despair happen to me. It doesn't have to be that way.

Even in the middle of deep isolation and frustration, though, she taught us to read, to ask questions, to look for answers. "What's this word, Mom?" I'd ask. "Sound it out," she'd say, instead of doing the easy thing — giving me the answer. "Break it down, take it bit by bit." Then she'd teach me the meaning of the Latin roots. From her, I learned to love language. And line, too: how many drawings did she make for me to color? — and then, when I got older, how many drawings did she help me make for myself? "Look closely," she'd say, when I was drawing a face. "See how the distance from the nose to the top of the head is the same as the distance from the nose to the chin." Later, years after I'd begun writing professionally, she set her jaw and told me, "Did we ever worry in this family about what other people might say about us? — You just write what you need to write."

I was probably the first kid in my class to have the Crayola set of sixty-four colors, with the built-in sharpener. She never liked to spend money, didn't even like to talk or think about money; but when it came to those two things, books and art, I could have almost anything I asked for — though I learned that a good child was a child who didn't ask for too much, too often.

Everywhere I go, he's going to go.

It's not like we're strangers to each other — he already comes with me everywhere. He's already been to so many places. At the Lyle Lovett concert the other night, I was wondering if he could hear the music. "We took you to hear this wonderful music before you were born," we'll say. Yesterday we took him to a friend's wedding at an African Methodist Episcopal church. I'll fly him to Maine next week ("Where did I put the tickets? — What's happening to me?"). We took him to Phoenix and the Grand Canyon in March. In January we'll take him to London. He'll see the world, not just the inside of his house, and not just from sitting in front of the tube. He'll see it firsthand. I hope he'll grow up feeling comfortable and confident moving from place to place. Traveling will be a way of life for him.

In childbirth class tonight we saw a video of three births. One was pretty quick, only four hours of labor, but the woman had already given birth twice. The other two were first-time moms, and one was in labor forty-eight hours before the baby finally came. Watching her breathe through thirty hours of contractions and never progress beyond three centimeters was exhausting and frightening. I can't imagine how it felt to go through it. Then after forty-four hours, she had to gather enough strength to push the baby out. I felt myself holding my own breath and wondered if, in her place, I wouldn't go ahead with the C-section.

We watched the baby's head tunneling through the pelvis, and I tried to imagine the pain. There's nothing smooth and streamlined about the maneuver: the baby squashed, the flesh of the labia stretched, like a vise holding the mouth open, with no relief. That woman who endured forty-eight hours of labor—her baby was born purple. "It's *purple*," the woman next to me whispered to her husband. It was: not pink or red but violet, as though it had withstood a good beating.

What if I can't do it?

After the video we all just sat there staring at the carpet. Sylvia asked us if it had made us feel better or worse about giving birth. No one even said anything for a minute, and then I said, "Worse," and the other two first-timers in the group just sighed.

Sylvia asked why. I said I was freaked out at the lack of control. The women you see in still shots of birth and the ones in tonight's video all look the same: whether they're draped across their "partners" or hung between two people on their "support team" or lying on their sides with one leg being held up, they all look out of control. Embarrassing, frankly. Totally vulnerable. Naked and and agonized, with nothing really helping them. At the mercy of this uncontrollable process overtaking their bodies. In uncontrollable pain.

They grunted, they groaned, they moaned in ways I imagine animals do when they give birth, or are about to die. They made sounds that I'm sure they couldn't duplicate without the concomitant pain.

Can I give myself up, lose myself in the process that way? Will I make it difficult for myself by refusing to surrender as much as my body needs to?

"There is nothing controlled about birth, is there?" Sylvia asked the woman in our group who is pregnant with her fourth. "No," the woman said. There isn't. She might have said *natural* birth. The only way you get total control over birth is to schedule a cesarean. If you want to feel your baby come out, then to some degree you have to surrender to the process that humans have evolved to push out their babies.

Judy has decided to pass on the childbirth classes. "We don't have time for them. Our schedules are totally insane, and classes would take up sixteen hours of time. Besides, we decided we'd just be totally bored."

"We practice a lot," I told her.

"Practice *what?*" she asked. Breathing, I said, and all the stuff that Nick's learning about how to help me relax during labor. But maybe none of that stuff will help, anyway. Maybe Judy needs a different kind of help. When I told Sylvia my sister's not taking classes, she said, "She'll probably be one of the first to have an epidural." OK, then — maybe that's the kind of help Judy needs.

♨

Two months and a day till due date.

Today the midwife said my uterus was thirty-one centimeters from pubic bone to fundus. The baby grew my uterus two centimeters in two weeks. Can my uterus really be more than a foot high? The midwife says he is about three pounds now, and he'll keep putting on about half a pound a week. But how can I get any bigger? — no matter which way I turn or how frequently I shift, my back hurts, especially between my shoulder blades and in the small of my back. When I hunch forward to stretch those muscles, my abdominals cramp, and I can't breathe.

I felt his head today. About the size of a small grapefruit. The size my uterus was at six weeks. "Here," the midwife said, pushing my fingertips into my pelvis just above my hairline, "you can slide his head back and forth between your hands. The head is the hardest part of his body — everything else feels soft and wiggly compared to the head."

I had Nancy again today. "Nancy the Midwife," the brass sign on her desk says. Swarthmore graduate; used to work at Hahnemann Hospital in Philadelphia, then in rural Delaware. Delivered one of Janey's girls. She's maybe a couple of years younger than I.

I was upset today after seeing the birth film at the childbirth class last night. I almost cried in her office. "I just don't know if I can do it," I told her, but that wasn't it. I know I can do it. I know I can get the baby out. It was the image of the women's labia separating, like swollen lips, separating as though they might split, and the women all the while naked and vulnerable, eyes open but not seeing, looking inward, into the pain. And the unearthly noises they made . . . how could I ever let myself make noises like that?

"It's interesting that you use the word *vulnerable* to describe women in labor," Nancy said. She has bright blue eyes, keen as a jay's, and a single blonde braid that falls down her back. "I always think of women in childbirth as powerful. I remember one woman giving birth who wore a red silk blouse. When I arrived, there she was, on her hands and knees on the bed, rocking back and forth in her red silk blouse." Last night Sylvia asked us to bring an object to the final class that would remind us of women's strength. "That red silk blouse made her feel strong," Nancy said. "That's why I like working here. I've worked in hospitals, and when the woman shows up, her own clothes are immediately stripped off and a hospital gown is thrown on her. Here, women can choose to wear whatever helps them."

When I finally admitted to her that what I'm afraid of is humiliating myself in front of other people, something unknotted inside me. I also admitted that I don't know what is happening to me. It's hard to cut through the fog in my head to the place where any meaning resides. I look back at all this time, since I took the pregnancy test on January 19, and it seems to me that until the end of March I was engaged in committing to this process, deciding that, yes, I will have this baby, I will do this pregnancy, I will consent to this idea. Only, it was an *idea*. It was still primarily an idea until about four weeks ago, at thirty-two weeks, when he started to get really big. From April through June I felt stoned on happiness, on that relinquishment of control, with no threat waiting around the corner. Each little discovery was a thrill — the sonogram, the movement, the bursts of energy — and I felt like a kid again myself, only happier, calmer, and more content than I'd ever been as a kid. And I had no physical discomfort, other than my growing belly, which presented no real problems. I had Nick's clothes, I bought big clothes, I was fine.

Then I got big, and the weather got hot, and I began to lose sleep. Turning over in bed began to be painful, and I had to pee every two hours. Then, two weeks ago, the muscles in my back and abdomen began to spasm, and now my emotional state has gone entirely downhill. My circulation is poor; my legs cramp when I stand too suddenly or try to walk the most modest of inclines; I'm clumsy and awkward and nearly fall over if I don't take care. "When I get up to pee at 3 o'clock in the morning," Judy said yesterday, "I lurch like Frankenstein." She's nearly six feet tall, but I know how she feels. In the middle of the night, I hold my belly with my hands like a thirty-eight-inch stoneware bowl that's going to slop over if I don't get to the toilet in time; it feels too heavy to be carried by my abdominal muscles alone.

Thirty-eight inches: that's what my waist measured Friday when Charlee last came.

Now I sometimes feel disgusted by the aesthetics of late pregnancy. Early on it was sensual; the bowl was small and rather voluptuous, one of the numerous undulations that were part of my woman's body, and

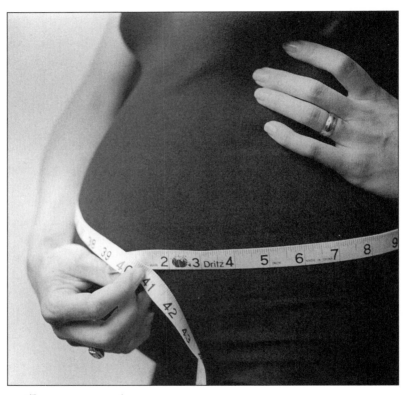

Twenty-nine weeks pregnant.

the little bowl taught me to appreciate my womanly curves. A couple of months ago, just by touching my belly during lovemaking, Nick could bring me to orgasm. But now it's a huge oven, like those big adobe domes the Pueblos build to bake their bread, and not at all sensual to me. It gets in the way.

Maybe he won't want to make love with me after seeing the baby born from between my legs. Maybe I'll wind up all stretched out. Maybe my breasts will become just feeding tubes.

Maybe when he sees the baby coming through me he won't be able to look at my body any other way anymore.

Maybe I won't be able to look at myself any other way anymore.

Oh God. What is happening to me?

"Birth will change you," Nancy said. "It will change the way you see your body. It will change the way you see yourself—it will make you grow into the new role of motherhood. It will change the relationship you have with your husband. You're not going to be the same after giving birth. *This is a big deal, here.*"

When I think about it, I just get tired and want to go to sleep. Except my body hurts so much I can't sleep.

What if I don't love him? What if he doesn't love me? The books even say that not all women feel like they love their babies as soon as they're born. Mom always said she didn't experience that. "I didn't feel that 'wave' of 'maternal love' people always talk about. Don't fall for that," she always said. "You can't love someone until you know who they are. I was just so *curious* about who you were."

Another scary thing: our choice to go to midwives. Nancy says only 6 percent of pregnant women in America choose midwife care; all the rest go to obstetricians.

"You better tell Mom you're having the baby at the hospital," Judy told me. "She said yesterday on the phone, 'You're having the baby in a *hospital*, right? — because I think Jenny's having the baby in some kind of *birth center* thing.' I told her they call labor and delivery buildings 'birth centers' now. But I think you should tell her again that you're going to the hospital."

"But she knows," I said. "I told Dad, and I *know* he knows it's a hospital, and I know he knows it's Allegheny General, because he asked me if that wasn't going to be a farther drive than Magee Womens Hospital. I told them."

"Yeah, well, you know how Mom is," Judy said.

I want a woman to be with me. That's what midwife means, after all — "with woman," someone to be with you through the crisis, the journey. The French word for midwife is *sage-femme* — wise-woman. It's what I want, but I become paralyzed with doubt: even though Grandma had midwife help with her seven babies (six, actually: the seventh time, she gave birth to my father by herself, before the midwife got there), I feel as though I'm grinding against the family and cultural grain with this choice.

"You are," Nancy said, lighting that bright, point-blank stare of hers on my face.

🤚

Portland, Me.

No one at this design school can believe I'm eight months pregnant. "You're the thinnest pregnant woman I've ever seen," said one of the students here. I'm *not* thin. I'm really healthy. People are used to thinking of pregnant women as pigs. Besides, how can I be "thin" when my belly is nearly forty inches? It's still not readily noticeable to people and I am wondering if "showing" means just plain getting fat. "Seventeen pounds is nothing," the student said.

"I was pregnant from here to here at eight months," said another student, whose kids are now sixteen and eighteen. She held one hand at neck level and the other at mid-thigh.

Nick said before I flew out that he thought my pregnancy would be "attractive" to the other students and not a put-off. He was right. There are more women than men, and they want to know if I've got a name for the baby, and are interested in hearing about the midwives, and in general lean over and listen to anything I care to say about being pregnant. It's so nonacademic, the perfect antithesis to talking shop.

❧

Tilden Pond, Me.

Nick met me two days ago in Portland with a rental car, and we arrived at our cabin on the lake yesterday afternoon. Now it's 8 A.M. and I'm enjoying another half cup of excellent tea and a bowl of muesli and local blueberries topped with yogurt. Breakfast is the only meal at which I can eat as much as I like without heartburn. By noon the heartburn always sets in.

Between Nick snoring, the kid kicking around inside me, and the chorus of frogs singing last night, I hardly got any sleep. Finally at 2:30 A.M. I took a Benadryl because I couldn't doze off. My back hurts and my head hurts in the morning; my shoulders hurt; my arms fall asleep when I curl them around a pillow, or else my legs cramp up if I flex or stretch the wrong way; my abdominals cramp up and I can't breathe, but then if I sit up straight my back hurts again. I'm simply miserable in my body. I can't find a comfortable position in which to write. I'm starting to think I may as well forget about writing for the next year, or possibly the next twenty-two years, until he starts paying his own bills. It's just the reality that mothers are the ones who make the greatest personal sacrifices. Look at Charlee's life. She loves it, but it's also a nightmare of time management.

Sometimes he kicks so hard that it's painful. Especially when he hits my ribs. I'm so short-waisted and he's so big that his bum is now squashed right up under my ribs. He's been head-down for six weeks or more, so it's his feet — his heels — jabbing my lower ribs. Pretty soon he'll kick me in the solar plexus. And he punches my bladder.

I've read that some women feel depressed after giving birth because they feel the loss of the intimacy of carrying the baby inside them constantly. On days like today, that statement makes me laugh. I think I'll just be relieved. I already feel some loss of intimacy because he's so big now that his movements feel less intimate, more attacking, as though he were trying to punch a tunnel through me so he can get the hell out.

Everyone thinks he's going to be late, even Nick, but I think he'll be early, a week, possibly two. I don't think he wants to wait around.

I don't always feel so angry and frustrated at him. I often like the company. Each day, I talk to him. When I go somewhere, I'll tell him where we are, what's going on around us. Last evening we took the canoe out onto the pond and I told him we were out on the water. I tell him Daddy's right next to him whenever Nick puts his face on my belly or puts his hands on my skin. Nick says this means I'm already forming a relationship with him, but does it mean that? It seems like playing with a baby doll might be more realistic. I don't even know what he looks like. I don't actually know what he's doing when he moves around; I'm only guessing. There are so many things I should do for him that I haven't done yet, like buying clothes and linens and toys.

I don't think we're going to find as much peace and quiet when we come up here next year with him.

☙

Tilden Pond.

Another difficult night sleeping, the bed is so hard. The rain seems to have gotten it over with during the night, and now the breeze smells of freshly watered balsam pine and the sky is a clear blue, with a few pure-white clouds.

I've found it hard to accept this downtime after such a frantic week at the workshop. I was much more wound up than I realized. I had almost no time to think and process what I was learning, but now my mind seems to be stretching out like a net and trying to hold thoughts and feelings. I've spent a lot of time here at the cottage just sitting and feeling grateful for my blessings, and of course suffering the crazy corollary fear that they will be taken away from me. Even now as I sit at the kitchen table watching the breeze ruffle the surface of the pond, the sunlight warming the soft carpet of pine needles under the picnic bench, listening to Nick cooking eggs and hash browns in the kitchen, I feel gratitude and right on the heels of that the question of when it will all go.

There's so much I can't control. That's what I'm still learning. I can't control how long Nick will be with me. I can't control the kind of personality our kid will have. I can't make the sun shine on our holiday.

I can tell I'm really getting near the end. I'm starting to have mood swings again, and I freak out, like I used to when I had PMS (having a period seems like another lifetime ago). I have moments of peace, but then my old rigid judgments and worries return.

Tilden Pond.

Last night in bed I told Nick all about these feelings. And as we talked I began to feel my body open up to his. We made love for a long time, and for the first time in two months I came, his face between my breasts. It was such a relief to me. I told him how deeply I'm committed to him, in an almost autonomic way. I trust him like I trust my ability to breathe, and I need him that much, and it makes me live. He said that it has happened for him as well. That he has no more doubts.

Tilden Pond.

Really struggling to keep the contentment I found during the calm second-trimester weeks. I focus on the small pleasures: we take the folding chairs down to the shore and plant them in the shallows. Tiny fish circle around our feet when we dangle them in the water, and we read together for hours in the silence under a constantly shifting cloudscape, pausing to enjoy the fresh breeze, the sun shafting down and splintering to diamonds on the far shore, the pair of loons fishing in early evening.

I returned the fifty-dollar bathing suit and, at my dependable discount store, bought a fourteen-dollar tank-style leotard that has shorts, and I wear this when I go into the water. Nick calls this excuse for a swimsuit my "late-nineteenth-century bathing costume" and chuckles appreciatively when I take down the straps to sun my shoulders.

Sitting by the pond in the sun, my skin browning, I felt so beautiful today. I don't think I've ever felt as beautiful in my entire life as I have the past few days. I like my big body, and I never expected to like it. As I look at our baby moving underneath the layers of skin and muscle in my belly, "swishing his bum," as Nick says, and see my breasts—huge, for being my breasts—with their nipples, now nearly black, that peak up at the slightest touch, I feel beautiful. Voluptuous. I forget which book says that pregnancy helps some women feel forever different and more accepting of their bodies. I think that will be me.

No matter what, though, I always end up thinking about the baby. Our little guy will see all of this next year. We can share everything we have with him.

We have a large extended family of friends who will love him. Von and Dale will love him. Jeri and Evelyn already call themselves "The Aunties." He'll have a cousin right away in Judy and Tim's baby, and

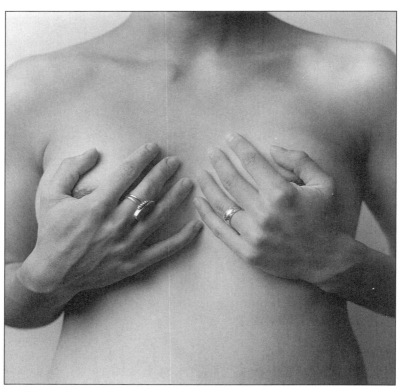

Thirty-five weeks pregnant.

uncle and aunt nearby in Joe and Claudine. My parents will love him, even dote on him. On *both* the babies.

I hope I can ask for the help we need after he comes. Nancy the Midwife urged me to do this at my last visit before I came away. I want him to belong to our little "village" at home. I don't want to keep him all to ourselves. I want him really to be "our baby" — all of ours.

Tilden Pond.

Spent our last full day here at the water's edge. A calm day today. Read down at the shore all afternoon today, watching the small fish circle my feet, and gulls coasting low over the mirrored surface, it was that easy for them to spot prey today. At noontime, five loons came out together to fish.

We leave tomorrow.

We'll have dinner in town, then a walk to the wharf to say goodbye for another year to the village we love so much.

The loons are calling their sad cry.

Nick reading a story I tore out of an old *U.S. News* at the laundromat: "Raising the Moral Child." "What about the intelligent child," he asked, "the happy child, the free child?"

Now ecstatic high warbling from the loons, and an occasional low moan from a frog.

In flight from Portland.

A wall of clouds is visible from my west-facing window — the cold front that will cool down the entire East Coast.

There's a screaming eighteen-month-old girl across the aisle whose parents are spending their whole reservoir of time and attention struggling to amuse and feed, to keep her quiet.

This is the most relaxed plane trip I can remember, and with the most baggage—two suitcases, two shoulder bags, a duffel bag, and a second-hand playpen packed into a carrier bag. I looked at it all this morning (in fact, I'd loaded most of it into the rental car, then sat down to breathe through ten minutes of contractions) and submitted to the knowledge that I could not carry it all—if any of it; I was not going to speed-walk through the airport, as I usually do; I couldn't be bothered to worry, as I usually do, about stuff breaking or getting lost. If USAir loses or breaks anything, I figure, they'll have to find or pay for it.

❦

Spent much of the day looking for supplies for the upstairs apartment renovation. Went to the kitchen place on Fifth Avenue and looked for wall-mountable cabinets in oak.

Nobody expects to see a woman so pregnant running around doing errands.

As a pregnant woman I am in an interesting social position. I'm highly noticeable and at the same time, paradoxically, I'm invisible. I attract attention—cracks, jokes—the kind of attention that doesn't help. And people remember me. I can walk into a store two days after I've just been there, and people will remember who I am because I'm "that pregnant woman." Or "that pretty pregnant woman"—not just any pregnant woman, not just any pretty woman. The combination seems to leave an indelible mark of the exotic, like a belly dancer walking into a Wall Street bank full of gray suits. I'm stared at everywhere and even am the butt of smartass comments — or else I'm pointedly ignored. Either extreme feels like an unhelpful response. I mean, I know I'm having mood swings, but my God, pregnancy is so common, you'd think people would want to help you instead of making fun of you! My belly seems like such a sign of my sexuality that people don't know how to respond comfortably. I had sex! It's like nobody can believe it. Or like nobody can believe I'm wearing such a sign of it. Are we supposed to hide the fact? I wish I had a T-shirt that said, "It Was Good for Me."

In the kitchen place I marched straight back to the room where they keep all the discounted returned merchandise. I'd seen a sales guy go back there already. He gave me an inquisitive look when I entered and I said, "I've been here lots of times — the receptionist said I could come back here."

"Of course, go right ahead," he said, turning to another guy in blue workpants holding a dolly. Then he turned back and added, with a smirk and a glance at my belly, "Don't trip!" I was in a dress, but it wasn't like I was wearing spike heels. I had my flat sandals on. "Don't worry about it," I said.

I found two floor-level cabinets, one in oak and one in hickory, which is a good match, plus an overhead oak cupboard. After some measuring and figuring on my part, I went to see the dealer, who said I could have all three for $150 — a better price than the unfinished cabinets we'd found the night before at Builders Square. And we wouldn't have to finish these. The dealer said they retailed for $900. I reveled in the money I was saving and in the image of them mounted on the wall upstairs. Coming back out from a final check, I almost bumped into the guy with the dolly, who was unloading large boxes from a truck parked at the dock.

"Gettin' your exercise this morning, aren'tcha?" he said.

"Yeah," I said, striding past him, "and I see you are as well."

He laughed. Then, as though not to allow me to have the last word, he called in a loud voice, "If you get tired, don't worry—I can just wheel you around!"

Like a crate to be dumped on a skid, I thought. Jeez. I kept walking. "No, thanks!" I called back.

God, am I that big?

Jeri says yes, though I've only gained twenty pounds. She skipped an afternoon of billable time for our foundation contracts (in the years I've worked for Jeri, I've learned how important it is to build in break time) and came with us to our prenatal appointment this afternoon, dropping by the house so we could drive over together. I was out picking beans, in the same yellow dress I'd worn to the kitchen place. The "lemon drop dress," Charlee calls it. "You're very big," Jeri said. But if I stand at a high counter and talk to someone, they can't tell that I'm pregnant. Sometimes they can't tell even when my belly's showing, if I'm wearing a big enough dress.

I wonder if it's because my appearance doesn't make people feel bad for me that I get such unhelpful, cheeky remarks from people.

Maybe I'm being just a *trifle* oversensitive?

Also, people don't move out of the way for me. Even though I don't look big, I am big, for me, and it's hard to maneuver myself in tight places. It's hard to hold myself upright for too long. The baby and his entire support system are heavy, and he's now big enough to pinch my sciatic nerve so that sometimes my right leg will give out and I'll nearly fall. Or my lower belly will seize up in a cramp, and I'll involuntarily bend double. Not once has anybody asked me if I'm OK.

But when I'm walking all right and looking attractive, they want to wheel me around like a load of inventory.

Also, people don't help me lift things. Except for Nick, who's constantly telling me I have to let him help me. This evening, while he hosted a meeting at the house, I was back at Builders Square to buy a six-foot precut Formica slab, plus an oak medicine cabinet and a ceiling fan. I had to ask the plumbing guy if he minded putting the medicine cabinet in the basket for me. He was going to hand this huge box to me, as though I weren't pregnant. Then I filled the rest of the basket with sundries—drywall screws, a toilet water-supply pipe, threshold trim, towel bars and TP holder, switch plates, all this stuff. Then I went to the lighting department to pick out a ceiling fan. I checked out the installation specs, and I called over a sales guy to help me figure out how large a fan to buy. I had to buy the largest one. "I guess I'll take this one," I said, pointing out a massive box holding a fifty-two-inch fan. I hoped the guy would lift it for me, but he just nodded. Couldn't he see I'm pregnant? He even stood there watching me as I groaned and heaved the box around my huge belly.

Now I know how handicapped people feel. Are you supposed to say, "Look, I'm *paralyzed,* I can't do everything by myself," when you're in a wheelchair? There's so little patience with people who move slowly or differently. Today in the elevator at the hospital I pressed the open-door button and watched as a woman struggled to push a guy in a wheelchair out of the elevator and through a crowd that had gathered to enter the elevator. Nobody moved — everyone just fixated on getting inside first, and this woman had to excuse herself half a dozen times before anyone took one step aside.

I couldn't fit the fan into the basket, so I put it on top of a stack of other fans and left my basket in the aisle next to the lighting department. Then I went to get the Formica slab.

Six feet of chipboard — sawdust and glue — laminated with Formica. I stood for fifteen minutes looking for endcaps in the correct color, while the kid punched my bladder and kicked my ribs, and everything else cramped. Finally I asked a saleswoman. "Looks like we're out of them," she said. "I can't even check for you to see if they're on order because the computers are down." So I had to just buy the slab, and hope I could find the caps in the right color somewhere else. What else could go wrong?

I asked her if there were any way someone could carry the slab to the front of the store. Eight months ago I could have hauled it myself. She told me it would be under the tent on display near the front.

A voice announced over the PA system that the store would close in twenty minutes. I lumbered back to the lighting department to retrieve my basket. But I couldn't find it.

Was it just pregnant-woman absentmindedness? I looked around, but no sign of my basket. I strode back to the Formica department, trying to ignore the stabbing in my belly, and looked in the bath and plumbing departments; no basket. By this time my spine felt like it might just split in half, a vine snapping under the weight of its fruit, and I was nearly in tears with fatigue and the heat. "Someone took my basket of stuff," I gasped to the woman behind the service desk, "and I need that stuff for tomorrow. It had a medicine cabinet in it." And drywall screws, and a water-supply pipe, and threshold trim, and everything else that would finish our job.

"Will the person who took the medicine-cabinet basket please bring it to the front of the store," she announced into the mike.

I dragged myself once more around stacks of light fixtures. Where on earth could I have put it? I was sure it was my own fault until I went back to the desk and saw the embarrassed look on her face. "They took that basket into the back," she said. "They thought the stuff was being stolen."

"Stolen!" I cried. "I spent *an hour and a half* gathering that stuff! And I'm eight months pregnant, and I can't drive a basket around the whole store! And you're closing in ten minutes! How will I ever get all that stuff back?"

Her eyes looked like they were going to pop out, and people were turning to look at me. I was making a scene. I have made scenes before, but always more or less deliberately, choosing my moment and language. This was coming straight out of some place I didn't know about, some place of spontaneity and belly cramps and bladder punches and total exhaustion.

And after all that, they only gave me a 10 percent discount!

♓

Jeri came with us to our prenatal appointment yesterday. She and I toured the midwives' new birthing rooms that are being built in one wing of the hospital. One of them has a huge freestanding Jacuzzi. All three rooms have Jacuzzis, in fact, but this one was big enough for two people. I wish I were going to be able to have the baby in one of the new rooms, but they won't be finished in time. Our appointment was with Kathy Evans-Palmisano, the center's director, who saw us for our first visit. She tried to convince me, ironically, that the new rooms would not help me in the least, and that many women prefer a shower to a tub because they can hold themselves upright more easily. "You know what? — when you're in labor, you don't give a damn *where* you are," she said, and her voice was really sympathetic and kind, but the statement begged the question of why they're spending hundreds of thousands of dollars on the new facility.

Nick didn't even want to see the rooms. "If we're not going to get to have the baby there, then I don't even want to know what we're missing," he said.

He and Jeri and I squeezed onto the loveseat in front of Kathy's desk. I was concerned that Jeri would feel weird at this particular appointment because we're at the stage where I have to start perineal massage, so I can avoid them needing to slice me up, and we needed

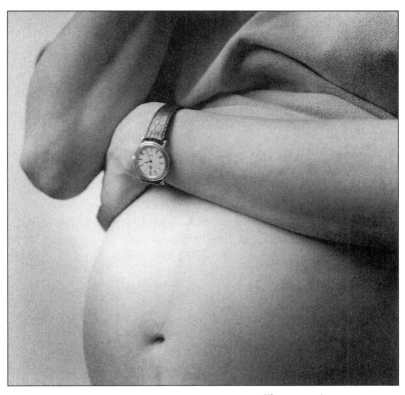

Thirty weeks pregnant.

advice on how to do that. "You need to get your fingers in the vagina pretty much up to the second knuckle," Kathy explained to Nick, "and massage in a U, then begin to pull gently until *you*"—looking at me—"start to feel a burning or stinging sensation."

"Does it really help?" I asked dubiously.

"I won't say it *guarantees* an intact perineum, but it does wonders," she said. Plus we were going to ask about breastfeeding, plus Kathy brought up the subject of sex in the last trimester. "Late-term lovemaking is fine," she said. "It is?" I retorted sarcastically, "I wouldn't call it 'fine.' "

I drafted our birth plan and made a copy for Jeri to read before the appointment. She'd stood in the kitchen reading it and asked, "Does breast stimulation actually promote uterine contractions?" One section of the plan talks about how Nick and I want to be able to touch each other in any way we want without feeling judged as inappropriate by the staff. Who knows what we'll want to do? But just in case, I asked, "Are the staff OK with physical contact?"

"Let me tell you a story," Kathy said. "I was at one woman's labor, along with the woman's husband, a nurse assistant, and a male midwifery student who was there to observe. The woman was using the sacral ball—we have this ball that women roll around on to relieve back pain during labor. This woman was moving around on this ball in such a sensual manner that even the midwife said she was getting turned on, just watching. The student said he'd never seen anything so sexy in his life. We *definitely* recognize the sensual aspects of labor."

Maybe it's just "hormones," but these mood swings are killing me. I feel like I need to have my period.

I'm having trouble working. My study is all torn up. I'm moving furniture in and out to make room for the crib in our bedroom. It's almost impossible for me to work when my study is a mess.

The kid has hiccups and it's making the notebook jump.

Nick's stressed out with the semester beginning soon. I feel as though I'm not doing enough to help. He has most of the burden of making money and now of doing the physical things around here, because I can't run around like I used to.

At least I'm not the only one who feels like she's going nuts. I visited Luisa yesterday in her remodeled kitchen. (We're all doing this "nesting." All the books say when you get to the last part of the third trimester, you start to "nest": rearrange furniture or redecorate rooms. Hoard little items for the baby. Judy's not just remodeling; she's moving into a whole new house.) "The contractor took twice as long as he said he would. July was a total drag. I haven't enjoyed this summer at all," Luisa said. She seems pretty unhappy. The mole on her forehead doesn't look to me to have grown much, but it's very visible and it gets on her nerves. I have trouble believing it can't be taken off just because she's pregnant.

She's even thinking that she doesn't want to have another kid because she has disliked this pregnancy so much. She's reluctant to breastfeed, which surprised me — nursing is without a doubt the best way to feed a baby. But "I just want my body back," she said.

"Luise, you can feed him for three months," I said. "Feed him for a month and let him get his antibodies and then switch."

"E.J. doesn't have an antibody in him and he never gets sick," she said. "We weren't breastfed and we didn't get sick. Did you get sick?"

"Yeah—I had pneumonia at eight weeks," I said, but that probably wasn't because I was a "formula baby." I was two weeks early, weighed only six pounds, two ounces. I was a quiet baby born into the late autumn, and Mom and Dad both smoked. Judy, on the other hand, had terrible respiratory allergies. They're even saying now that nursing prevents allergies and asthma. Our generation's mothers got suckered into the formula ad campaign, the same one that killed third-world babies. I read all about it in Rothman's book. People used to boycott formula manufacturers because of it.

"Besides," I said, "I just think nursing's going to be convenient. I don't want to have to go out and buy bottles and formula and drag around one of those huge bags just to feed him. I want to put him in a sling and go walking around the city and when he gets hungry just find a ladies' room or a quiet corner and feed him."

"That's *another* thing," Luisa said. "I don't think I can just whip it out like that, you know what I'm saying? My cousin has no problem just whipping it out, even on the street—"

"But she's in Italy, and grew up there, right?"

"Yeah," she sighed.

"So you find a ladies' room," I said. "Or you get used to it."

"I *can't* get used to it," she said. "I'm huge, and I'm going to have boobs out to *here* soon—"

"They're not going to get any bigger at this point, Luise," I said. We're at the end of our eighth month.

"They're *going* to get bigger, because right now they don't have anything in them!" she exploded. "Jen, you're so small, so you don't have to worry."

"Luise, I'm *not* small, I wear a 38 bra now."

"What size cup?" she demanded. She would not give up.

"B," I said, "but pretty soon it's going to be a C," discarding the idea that they wouldn't get any bigger.

"I'm into a *D*," she said flatly, throwing out her hands, "I've *crossed that threshold*, and it just *depresses* me. I *can't* get any bigger! I can't do it!"

E.J. walked in. "I think I've got this crib figured out," he told Luisa. He asked me how I'm feeling.

"You look like you're going to pop," Luisa told me. "You look like you've gotten a lot bigger."

"So do you," I said.

"No, I don't," she said, "not as big as you."

"What do you think, E.J.?" I stood next to Luisa.

He shrugged. "You both look about the same," he said. The diplomatic father-to-be. He went back upstairs to finish putting the crib together. Luisa watched him go and sighed.

"This baby isn't going to come soon enough for me," she said.

"Luise," I said, meeting her eyes, "this is *happening* — "

"I know," she said, shaking her head.

" — we're having babies."

"I know."

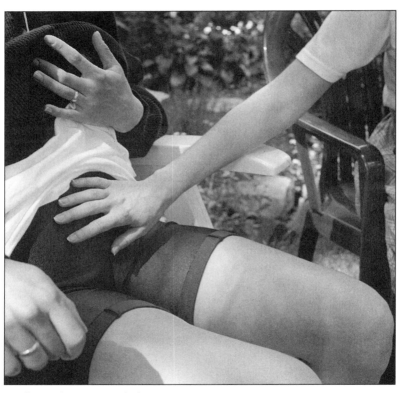

Luisa feeling our baby.

I sound so sure of myself when I talk to Luisa or Judy, but when I'm alone my bravado breaks. I have never faced so much uncertainty and it's driving me crazy. Everything would be so much easier if I knew the baby were absolutely OK; if I knew what sort of personality he has; if I knew what kind of apartment we'll have when Nick begins teaching in London in five months; if I knew exactly when the baby is going to come, preferably what day, and what hour of the day; if I knew who's going to be living in our third-floor apartment while we're in London, and how much they're going to pay; and if I knew who's going to take care of the cat while we're in London. If I knew all this, I could plan exactly how much money would be coming in and going out, how much time I could devote to work (both paid and unpaid), and the tenor of our lives during the next nine months — till we get back from London. As it is, I am paralyzed by the lack of knowledge, the lack of possibility even to venture an educated guess, about any of these factors, which are usually so stable and predictable. To calm my nerves I sit and read *Sister Carrie* or some other novel I've read a million times before, consoling myself with dense, highly organized nineteenth-century prose and the sense that other people exist, if "only" in literature, who are more out of control of their lives than I.

I can't believe it — we may have found a person to live in our apartment upstairs while we're in London. Not a graduate student, but the new CEO of a social service agency with a $15 million budget and a staff of 450. In other words, somebody smart and responsible.

I really needed that jolt of synchronicity to keep me going.

I feel hungry all the time, but I also feel nauseated. It's the lack of control. The further I go along, the more I assume I'll *gain* control. Do I really think that, once he's born, things are going to get *easier* to manage? Each step of the way, the more control slips away from me, and I have to keep learning to let go and trust.

❦

It's 6 A.M. and I've given up trying to get some sleep. I always feel horrible in the morning. A month and three days till due date: I don't want to believe that I have *five more weeks* of this left. Everybody says I'll be even more tired after he comes. I hope that after he's born I'll be *able* to sleep when I lie down. Now, when I lie down, I can't breathe and I can't move. Each time I get back up, I end up thinking I should call a heavy equipment place and rent a crane for this last month.

In the last two days I've been freaking out over having to quit work. The three writers—including myself—who work for Jeri met at her house for a planning session two days ago. There we are, sitting around the table, I've got my elbows propped on the edge and my belly hanging under my arms. They're all wearing suits and jewelry, and I've got on my nineteenth-century bathing costume with a T-shirt over it. Jeri asks me to talk about my work schedule for the next six months and everyone turns to me. "Well," I venture, "I'm scheduled to have a baby in about five weeks." Everyone laughs, but I'm serious: he could be two weeks early or two weeks late. It would be so much easier to feel sane if I knew when he is coming—if I had a window of arrival narrower than four weeks.

Here's an example of the way I schedule my life lately: Jeri and I were hoping to receive a story list for a client newsletter yesterday, but it's clear they may not give us one for another week or two. Which may or may not cut me out of that work. If they get us the list in one week, and I'm a week or two late (as *everybody* says I will be), I might be able to crank it out. If they wait two or more weeks and I'm a week or two early, then the work falls on Jeri's head.

I feel like I'm letting the team down and sticking them with extra work. Maybe they'll get so comfortable with the people who are going to sub for me that they won't want me back when we return from London. Jeri says she doesn't even have an inkling of not wanting me back. We've got a three-year working relationship and a nine-year friendship under our belts. That's a lot of trust — in each other and in our professional process. Jeri talked about how she wants the business not only to provide money but also to support our emotional lives and our need for interdependence. For me, it already does that. I couldn't imagine a better work situation.

The meeting lasted three hours, but it didn't seem a bit tedious. I left with the same sense of support that I get during my checkups with the midwives. Both teams support the whole woman — not just her wallet, not just her reproductive system.

I might be the only one of us who's looking forward to nursing. Judy told me today that she's feeling reluctant to breastfeed. "I've been reading all about it," she said, "and no matter what way you cut it, it's a lot like being a cow. It's very animalistic, every part of it." The only aspect of it that gives me the creeps is the idea of expressing my milk. A breast pump seems so mechanical. Maybe there's another option I don't know about.

Among all the massive changes that have occurred in my body, the most shocking for me is the functionality of my breasts. One day at Tilden Pond I stepped out of the hot shower and squeezed my right breast just to see what it would do. I didn't really expect to see anything, but a drop of yellowish milky fluid seeped out. I felt a pang in my belly—excitement ("They work!") and disgust ("I'm a cow"). I walked into the kitchen and showed Nick, who just smiled. "Aren't you shocked that my breasts work?" I asked him. "No—but you *want* me to be, don't you?" he teased.

I'm slightly suspicious of this new utilitarian role for my breasts. But I also believe feeding the baby with my breasts will be one of the healthiest things, both physically and emotionally, that I could ever do for him. Feeding a whole person with my own body—I try to imagine it. He's going to need me and feel close to me when I feed him, and I'm going to let him feel that way and give him the food and attention he needs, and hope that somehow my feelings will sort themselves out enough to permit me to do it.

Judy and I compared notes about our latest doctor's visits. I told her I was disappointed because my fundus was only thirty-three centimeters high, one centimeter short of the average height at thirty-four weeks. Nancy the Midwife said (of course) that it's not a problem.

"You know how big your uterus is?" Judy said.

"The midwife always tells me after she measures me. Doesn't your doctor measure you?" I said.

"Yeah, but he never tells me what it is."

"But don't you ask?"

"No: I just say, 'Is it OK?' and he says yes. Hopefully."

Even at nearly nine months, my pregnancy remains largely hidden. Getting my hair cut yesterday, I was draped with a nylon robe, and no one could tell I was eight and a half months pregnant.

I was desperate for a radical haircut. I'm so tired of the way I look. My hair is growing so fast now — it got shaggy in just five weeks. The books say with pregnancy's increased metabolism, your hair and fingernails might grow faster. I was ready to ask for a punk cut, spikes on top, color streaks or *something* — I didn't know what. "Do something to make me pretty, Joe," I whined.

"I have three or four clients all about eight or nine months pregnant. You've all come in recently with the same line — 'Do something to make me pretty,' " he said. "It's like you all see yourselves as looking really *different*, but to me you look the same, just pregnant." He moved in on my bangs and snipped them less than an inch long before I realized what the hell he was doing. "He couldn't be cutting me that short," I thought, in direct contradiction to the evidence in the mirror.

Then Joe's orange Polo shirt with the blue man-on-the-horse came between me and the mirror and I gave up, closed my eyes, and just listened to Joe talk. "My one client, she's about as far along as you, she's *really conservative* — I mean, she's a doctor, she used to be on the president's board of physicians in D.C. — she came in not too long ago and asked me to make her a blonde. I said, *'Sharon, you're* not *a* blonde.' She said, 'Yeah, I thought you'd say that, so why don't we do some streaks instead? I need something *radical.'* So I put in some streaks. I just know she's going to come in here after she has the baby and say, 'Why did I do this?' " He sighed as he snipped. "And I'll have to make her a brunette again. Luckily, with just the streaks, I won't have too much damage to fix.

"This baby was a surprise for her, too," he said. "She's, like, thirty-eight or thirty-nine. She was telling me how, now that her kids are getting big, she and her husband were getting ready to move back to D.C., and then one day she comes in and says, 'Joe — I'm *pregnant.'* " He sighed again. "I was like, *'Sharon,* I know how, but *how?* — you're both *doctors!"*

"Technology is not infallible," I said. "Believe me."

"I guess not," he said, laughing and stepping behind me to reveal a haircut so short and sweet that I could be Audrey Hepburn in 1959, I could be Winona Ryder, I could announce videos on MTV, except that I am over thirty and eight and a half months pregnant. Maybe they could shoot me from the shoulders up, like Elvis.

"Pretty girl," said another stylist, passing behind Joe. She was about my mother's age and dark, with black hair pulled into an Evita-style chignon. She could have looked Cuban but because this was Pittsburgh I knew her family had come from southern Italy.

"I can't be a girl anymore," I said, "I'm almost nine months pregnant."

"Oh, you're *pregnant?*" she exclaimed, and, peering into my face, pronounced, "You're going to have a boy."

"I am going to have a boy," I said.

"You see, I was right!" she said. "I knew right away."

"What are you *talking* about," Joe cried.

"Look at her—her complexion's beautiful," she said. "When you're having a boy, your skin clears up, you can't even get a pimple. With girls, your skin's a mess. When I was pregnant with my son," she said, turning her tanned face to me, "I *glowed.*"

"That's all such *crap!*" Joe cried again.

"It's the truth! And here's another way you can tell, this is how they tell in Sicily, my aunt from Sicily did this to me: I was driving in the car, I had my hands on the wheel, like this," she said, grasping an imaginary steering wheel, "and she asked me, 'How'd you get your hands so dirty?' And I looked at my hands like this," she said, holding her hands out palms down. "And if I would have held them like this," she said, turning her palms upward, "it would have meant I was having a girl. But because I did it the other way, I was having a boy."

"*Where* do they get these *stories?*" Joe said.

"I couldn't even tell you were pregnant," she said to me. "Boys you carry only in front, girls you—"

"You carry all over," I said. "Yeah, right."

Later, when Joe finished with his brushes and gel and gave me the hand mirror so I could see the back, two guys he works with stood admiring my new cut, nodding with appreciation at Joe's skill. Joe unsnapped the robe and I heaved myself out of the chair. "Oh, she's *pregnant!*" one of them said.

What am I supposed to say? My hand involuntarily fiddled with the cowlick at the back of my neck as I returned their stares.

"I just couldn't tell, that's all," he said.

As I stepped to the cash register I realized that, the next time I got my hair cut, I'd no longer be pregnant. I'd be a mother.

"Good luck with, you know, *everything,*" Joe said as I handed over my credit card.

✋

Not sleeping deeply anymore. Last night I had a better night's sleep than in days, but I never seem to get down into deep sleep. I just float on top, no matter how exhausted I am.

I think we've finally sorted out our furniture situation. The mahogany dresser that's been mine for ten years is now Nick's; the short oak one he bought four or five years ago is now mine, and in my study. The crib is in our bedroom, piled with the things given to us by family and friends. The crib doesn't belong in this room and will only stay here until we get back from London, when it will move into the room across the hall. The issue of where the baby is going to sleep is a question that's more freighted with pediatric analysis and cultural prejudice than I ever imagined. Some people argue that human evolution makes it "natural" for human babies to sleep next to their parents and point out that, in indigenous cultures, the kids sleep with their parents for years. Other people say that's all well and good for tribes of hunter-gatherers who sleep in the bush, but living in postindustrial society comes with the advantage—or the baggage, depending on how you look at it—of not having to protect your sleeping baby from snakes or wolves. Dr. Spock (whose book Von and Dale gave us) has a whole section called "Out of the parents' room by six months if possible," in which he says right off that newborn babies can (meaning "should") sleep by themselves. All these people are correct, of course. I don't know how we're going to decide what to do. I guess we'll just try to let intuition guide us. Right now it's telling us that we want him in the crib, but in the room with us. Who knows how we'll feel once he's born.

We've been given so many lovely things for the baby. "The Aunties" gave us a lambskin for his crib; another friend handmade a crib-sized quilt. Mom crocheted a butter-colored sweater and bootie set and a white crib afghan. I think back to that time I worried why she didn't ask about our baby: she must have been crocheting these beautiful things even then.

I'm slightly intimidated by all these little clothes. I guess I haven't exactly been relating to this kid in a practical way. Yet he's getting bigger and more independent all the time. He moves with increasing authority, as though he's really made my belly his house, and is becoming impatient with how small his quarters are.

The progressive bodily changes drag my attention away, out of my head and into my body. My breasts hurt all over again. I blow my nose, my forearms press against my chest, my nipples leak onto my shirt. Something—hormones, probably—is telling my body that it's almost time. Hormones are powerful chemicals, and the physical and psychological changes they produce are mysterious and startling. My breasts produce liquid food. They function. All so suddenly, without a word of permission from me. They begin their work silently, and I must learn how to facilitate it. I can't put it off. I can't say, I'll learn all about it *later*. They function *now*. It's not a fax I can leave on my desk for a few days.

♨

Despite all the worrying I do in here, I've been happier and more content in my pregnancy than I've ever been in my life. And having Charlee's pictures to look at week after week has helped me come to accept my body more than I could have done without them. It has changed my relationship with my body permanently. When I told this to Nancy the Midwife today, she said, "And the way your body is in relation to the rest of the world." Which is true. Look at our choice to go with the midwives. That's a choice that affects my body's relation to the rest of the world. I've been building a real relationship with our caregivers so I can rely on them in the extreme pain of childbirth. That's because I want to feel the labor as much as I can, and not numb my body out. Opting for no anesthetic is enough to produce some anxiety. Doing it with no doctor and none of the hospital apparatus that everyone else has — IVs, fetal monitors, epidural catheters, the works — sometimes makes me think I'm crazy. Then I think about Grandma and how she had seven babies at home, with no doctor; and I think of all the women all over the world who have relied on other women to help them through labor; and I know that I want to do it this way.

"Jen's going the *all-natural* route," Luisa told the women at her shower yesterday, and some of them groaned.

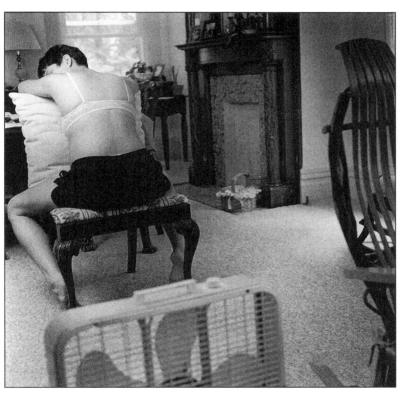

Thirty weeks pregnant.

They were sharing their labor stories. "Sometimes it takes them forever to get the epidural ready," one woman said. This woman has two kids, the second just seven months old, and I was interested in hearing her advice. "What you do is, when you go in for admission and they ask you your name, you say, 'I'm Kathy *Epidural.*'" The others laughed. "If you say it right away, you won't have to wait so long. I'm a baby about pain."

There were lots of murmurs of assent around the group, and Luisa laughed and said, "I'm having every drug known to man," and it hit me again that Nick and I have chosen the road less traveled—at least in this country. In most other countries, midwives are the "normal" route.

"I think we mostly get women who want more choice and control over pregnancy and childbirth," one of the birth center nurses told us today. My priority is to keep myself open to the experience, to get help in working through the pain, rather than trying to escape it. As "Kathy Epidural" was talking, a picture of myself arose in my mind, a woman in a blue hospital gown, a needle in her arm, catheters in her back and in her urethra, her feet up in stirrups, a masked doctor standing between her legs informing her that her baby had just been born. What a rip-off. For me, at least.

Maybe that's not the way it would be, after all. Maybe "the all-natural route" is going to be just a bunch of self-inflicted torture. I don't know *what* to expect. In my least confident moments I pore through the books that tell you what to expect, as though I will find The Answer. I do find a lot of answers, along with a lot of patronizing advice and silliness. Take a shower to relax during early labor, the experts write, "but be careful not to slip." Like the guys in the kitchen store wanting to wheel me around on a dolly.

"Why are you reading those books?" Nancy cries. "Throw them away!" A moment later she says encouragingly, "I think you'll pleasantly surprise yourself."

The false sense of certainty of the experts only unnerves me and makes me feel less confident than ever, less able to trust my physical and emotional experience. Invariably I wind up flinging the book in a corner of our bedroom and curling up on the bed, depressed. If your baby moves in a "panicky" way, they say, "call your practitioner immediately." Was the way he kicked before I ate lunch today "panicky"?

"Does it mean he's having a seizure?" I ask Nancy. She just rolls her eyes.

🖐

Nick sent the final payment in six years of payments to his ex-wife this week. No more ties to her. And just a month before our baby is due to be born.

The same day, we sat at dinner in a restaurant, and as we looked at each other and held hands, something opened up in his face and made me ask, "What do you *really* want to name him?"

"Jonathan," he said immediately, and as he said it, it felt right.

"Why?"

His eyes grew wet and I knew he was thinking of his brother, ten years younger than he. All his family still live back in England, and we see them only once a year. "Because I love him," he said, his voice thick.

"OK," I said. It's decided, as simple as that.

Judy sounds pretty eager for the whole thing to be over. She's got a rash all over her legs and belly. It gets worse at night and keeps her awake. She's tried hydrocortisone and antihistamine creams but nothing helps. Even taking two Benadryl capsules every four hours doesn't stop the itching or even make her sleepy. Adrienne Rich had the same reaction late in her first pregnancy. It sounds as though, as Rich wrote, Judy's "allergic to pregnancy." They're talking about inducing her, since the baby is nearly thirty-seven weeks. Judy said, "I can't do this for another six weeks," which is how long it could be before her labor begins naturally (but only if she were to be extremely late). When I called last night to tell her we'd be visiting, she sounded so tired — of everything, probably, of moving house and not having time or energy to unpack, of insomnia and itching, *everything.*

I haven't slept for the past two nights. Our waterbed has become uncomfortable, and I haven't found a way to arrange the pillows around my belly and back to make it possible for me to sleep without stabbing pain. I wake every hour, not to pee but to shift and allow blood to circulate to my limbs. Last night at 3 A.M. I finally got out of bed, dragging one pillow with me, and stumbled to the living room, where I sat on the couch, crying, feeling totally depressed at the prospect that I would never sleep again. I'm so desperate for sleep. I've never felt this way before. I'm *always* able to sleep. I even sleep in places like planes and cars and buses. Once, during a four-hour lay-over in Gatwick Airport, with hordes of people from all over the world and guards with machine guns milling around, I had a sound nap. Now

I understand how Nick has felt all these years when he wakes in the middle of the night unable to sleep.

♆

Up in the middle of the night again after waking from a dream: Nick and I were hiking a high trail in the forest. We ran into a couple from our childbirth class, and in the dream their baby had died. I don't remember anything else about the dream except that the trail was silent and beautiful but lonely, and the woman was still in deep grief, but they seemed to be having a cheerful walk. Feeling haunted by the tone of the dream.

Maybe my irregular sleep has distorted my sense of proportion, or maybe my energy level has me down. Whatever it is, I'm so bothered that I came downstairs an hour ago and sat reading Dr. Spock and eating hot fudge topping out of a jar, like a depressed teenage girl, until I realized what I was doing and threw the jar in the trash. Now I'll have a sugar crash.

I feel as though I've spent most of my life being pregnant. I forget what it was like to be alone, not to have this wiggling ball stuck to the front of me all the time.

Luisa said Thursday that she's going to try to breastfeed after all.

I'm so tired. Have I said that already? In case I haven't made it perfectly clear, let me say that I am *soooo* tired. It's nearly 5 A.M. and I've been up for ninety minutes and now I'm going to try to sleep on this couch. It seems to be the only place that's at all comfortable. I hate that I can't sleep with my husband.

I miss making love with Nick. When I no longer have this huge belly, I'm going to make love with him every day.

Only twenty-four days left. And maybe less.

Up at 3:30 this morning and dragged myself to the couch again. My lower belly was too sore to sleep in bed. The waterbed has come to feel like an instrument of torture. It never lets me drop off to sleep — I have constant stabbing all over my body. Like settling down for a nice nap in the Iron Maiden. It doesn't matter how tired I am. I busted my butt two days ago on the house and in the garden, hoping I could wear myself out so I could get five straight hours of sleep. Instead, my lower belly was so sore it kept seizing up, and my thighs ached from so much squatting. Instead of just tiring me out and letting me sleep, it tired me out *and* kept waking me up.

Here we sit in bed at 8 A.M. with baby stuff strewn on the floor waiting to be washed. "I want to be the one who stays home and does the laundry," Nick said as he watched me separate the whites out. He's going into the office all day and I'll stay here, bidding out a bunch of print jobs, finishing a catalog layout, washing baby paraphernalia, setting up interviews, cleaning the hall bathroom, tidying the front hall for our new tenant, and hopefully finishing all this in time to make dinner. Nick can have it — I'd rather go to the office, but this is where I am today.

I'm one week into my ninth month tomorrow. Twenty-one days left.

I cry every day, out of panic, at the unknown trial of labor and the prospect of taking care of such a little tiny person.

A good stroller — one that's light, sturdy, and can fold to fit on a plane or train or bus — costs at least $129.

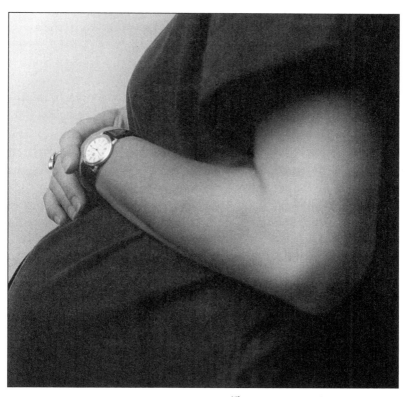

Thirty-seven weeks pregnant.

Here I am, whining, when I have it so much better than so many other people. How many pregnant women have husbands who *want* to stay home and do the laundry? Who *want* to stay home with the kid? I have more stuff going for me than I habitually acknowledge. More strength inside myself, more support, even more supplies. Sorting everything into laundry piles this morning, I saw clearly that we have more than enough stuff. Still, because I feel so emotionally unprepared, I feel compelled to get more. It's just a feeling, but it drives my actions, drives my speech, drives me crazy.

Sometimes I really envy Judy. I wish I were as sensible and practical as she is. She just faces a problem and tries to solve it, and doesn't get bogged down with all the feelings. In fact, she ignores the feelings. To her, they just get in the way of solving the problem. I remember telling her I think feelings have to do with every major decision in life, and she told me she thinks they're irrelevant. We were talking about choosing and closing on their new house. "That has nothing to do with feelings," she said. "That's purely a financial problem." As though debating about money has nothing to do with feelings about money. She decides: OK, I'll try washing our own diapers; I won't feel badly that my husband can't/won't help me, it's the reality of being married to a doctor; if it takes too much time, I'll switch to disposable diapers, and I won't feel guilty for polluting the environment. That's life. Deal with it.

I'm just not built that way. I have to say or write what I'm feeling, or I might as well climb into a *straitjacket.*

We went up to Cleveland yesterday to visit Judy and Tim. Their house is a four-bedroom ranch. It's a nice place, with nearly half an acre. She showed me the baby's room. There was a flannel nightshirt for the baby and an afghan—crocheted by my mother. Mom gave her the crib my grandfather made by hand before my mother was born. It's oak or maple or some beautiful hardwood. All the joints are pegged, and a brass plaque on the end is engraved with his name and the date: 1941. I was a little jealous, but only a little, and it was fleeting. I found his crib on my own; his mother and father chose it together.

Judy looked better than I had expected. She's gained some extra weight in her arms and shoulders, but her face looks the same as before she was pregnant, only she's pale from not being able to sleep. Her ankles are another story. The rash is the color of raspberry purée. Her toes are puffy and the skin is sewn with swollen veins around the ankle bones.

"Will it go away?" I asked.

"After delivery," she said.

"It'll all be gone within two weeks after," Tim said.

"Two *weeks!*" she shrieked. "I thought they said two *days!*"

As we sat in the kitchen and they each ate two pieces of the peach pie I'd brought them, every few minutes she'd uncap a tube of prescription hydrocortisone cream and dab a dot of it on some itchy patch.

"Look at your ankles," she said accusingly.

"What about them," I said.

"They're *normal ankles,*" she said. Her legs are so swollen that they follow a straight line from her calves to her heels.

They gave us a cute little outfit and a miniature soccer ball—for the soccer player in Nick. "In Pitt colors, of course," Judy said. And I think they really liked the stuff I made. She exclaimed over the teddy bears on the blanket and nearly teared up at the ladybug buttons on the sleeper.

I realized I put on a lot of bravado, I guess as compensation for how weak and scared I am feeling. Nick is at me every day to ask him to help me, but I keep thinking I can do everything by myself. Or that I *should* do. As we were wishing each other good luck with our labors before leaving, Judy said, "You'll be fine."

"Hmm, I don't know; I hope so," I said.

"That's the first uncertain thing that you've said today," Tim said.

"The truth is," I said, "I'm scared shitless."

☙

When the sun goes down I feel immobilized, isolated, out of control. I cry every night. It's a huge, sobbing cry that shakes my body and leaves me drained. Part of it is the knowledge that I'll go to bed and never reach a deep sleep. I wake every ninety minutes with a cramp in my lower belly or groin. I heave myself painfully out of the waterbed—like vaulting over the side of a swimming pool while wearing a lead life-saver. Lying still for any period of time *hurts*. Without my normal eight hours it's so trying to my temper and my body. I have a headache every day again and I am back to the daily struggles: over whether to take medication, over my dwindling temper, over fears that swarm in my brain when my strength is down.

I love to sleep. As long as I get eight continuous hours, I feel good when I wake up.

Nevermore, quoth the raven.

Will I ever sleep again?

"The worst thing was the not being able to get sustained sleep," Mom said ominously when I called her Saturday. "You ate every three hours. You were a small baby — six pounds, two ounces; Joey was bigger, seven-eight, and he ate every four. Finally I negotiated with your father that he would take the Saturday night feeding so that I could get one full night of sleep. I can't tell you the difference that made."

But I'm going to nurse. Nick says that's no reason he can't help. "If you *didn't* let me help, I'd fight you," Nick says.

"But you have to work."

"But you need to rest."

"But Judy's and Luisa's husbands aren't going to get up and bring the baby to them."

But, but, but. "How do you know that? *You don't know what other people are going to do!*" he says. Which is true, I can hear Helen agreeing.

"But my mother told me . . ."

His eyes instantly revert to the paper. "Sometimes I think your mother is like Mount Rushmore to you — huge, and carved in stone."

Despite the headaches that I get up with each day, the mornings are bearable again. There's a sense that everything's possible at 6 A.M. — I have so much time. As the clock winds toward 2 and there's so much left undone, so many problems have cropped up, and my energy wanes and my heartburn sets in, I just want to sit down and put my feet up and read, but the load of work and my compulsiveness about getting it done won't let me. Yesterday, I washed all the baby's clothes and linens, running (yes, sometimes running) up and down the stairs between the laundry and my study. I unwrapped pacifiers and baby nail clippers and bottles of ipecac, stocking the medicine cabinet, alternately taking business calls and folding clothes tinier than I've ever handled (sometimes tinier than I've ever seen: can any human being be so tiny?), alternately faxing out quote requests for print jobs and taking return calls from diaper services. I know the compulsion to do it all and do it perfectly comes from Mom, but at this point, knowing that doesn't seem to make a difference in the way I behave.

"Maybe in the coming weeks you might think about the kind of mother you'd like to be — the kinds of things you see yourself doing differently from your own upbringing," Nancy the Midwife suggested last week.

"I've sort of begun to do that," I replied, but have I? Have I made the time? I'd love to make the time. It seems too luxurious. "When you get to the last month," Janey told me back in January — eight months ago — "you'll just relax and lie in bed letting Nick give you footrubs, reading baby-name books and waiting for the baby to come." I'm waiting for the baby to come but I have not yet put up my feet to be rubbed. I can't imagine it. In my mind, "mother" is always rushing around doing things for other people — not taking it easy; not taking care of herself, much less letting other people take care of her. I know Mom wasn't that way all the time; but I can't think of a time when she allowed us to take care of her. That refusal to let others take care of me is one part of her character that's deepest in me. One thing I'd like to *try* to do differently is go a little more easily on myself.

🖐

It's the middle of the night. I can't sleep, so I'm downstairs on the couch reading and listening to the crickets sleepily cheeping outside. The window is open only a crack because it's falling into the 40s tonight — only 65 to 70 today. Perfect weather for jeans and a sweater. I long to put on a pair of blue jeans, a clean T-shirt, and a wool sweater and go for a crisp walk.

I look at the pictures of pregnant women in *Our Bodies, Ourselves*, remembering seeing them when I was ten weeks pregnant and feeling huge but thinking, "I'll never get that big." I was so small then. I am now in fact that big.

In the middle of the night, I sit and wait. "It's like waiting for Christmas when you're little — you never know when it's going to come," Judy said. And it seems so long, the waiting. It's like waiting for a visitor who's going to stay permanently, and you don't know when he's going to arrive, I told Evelyn this evening.

We're all waiting. "I just want it to be *over,*" Luisa says. "But then I think, 'Oh my God, what am I going to do when it *comes?*'"

"Are you afraid?" Evelyn asked me. I'm terrified.

I leave Nick sleeping in bed. His face looks so peaceful and smooth in sleep, or near-sleep. Suddenly I'm afraid he'll die. "Don't leave me," I whisper. "I ain't leavin' you, Babe," he mumbles from the brink. I kiss his forehead and slip out of bed (really I heave myself out) to let him sleep.

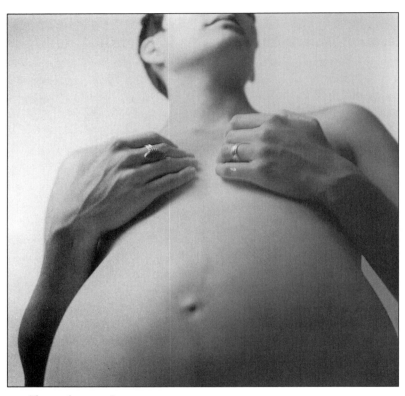

Thirty-five weeks pregnant.

Part of feeling emotionally low is my physical depletion, my inability to sleep, exercise, or even walk without pain. A brisk walk might clear my mind.

I wake, and I don't know what day it is anymore. Day and night have merged. I don't sleep well in the night; I catnap in the day.

Lighten up!

Looking at the rain this morning, I remembered I dreamed last night that it was raining and producing a rainbow, a small one hanging so low that I could touch it, put my hand into it from where I stood in our back yard.

In Rothman's book about "women and power in the birthplace," a midwife says her birth center tries to "create a milieu that is safe and supportive in which individuals can discover for themselves what it means to give birth. To open themselves on physical, emotional and spiritual levels to another person—to give birth."

Opening. Giving birth.

Our birth center handbook advises partners not to shout "Push!" during second-stage labor, but rather to encourage the woman to "open."

When Nick massages my perineum, as he's been doing every other day for three weeks, I can feel that it's a tight ring of muscle. It contracts itself—closes—when I'm upset or wound up—which is most of the time these days. As he stretches the tissue, I take a deep breath, exhale, and send a gentle signal along my spine to *open.* And it does. The subtlety of the experience reminds me of the way Stephen

Mitchell explains the Taoist practice of *wei-wu-wei* — "doing not-doing." Opening is not-closing. Opening doesn't mean forcing it open, but letting it not-close.

Soon I must open to this other person living inside me. I must let him move through me and try not (or not-try) to hinder his passage. I have to be the conduit. Right now I'm the container, and soon I'll be emptied out.

🖐

Tried sleeping in the spare bed in Nick's study. It worked better than the waterbed but it's so hard that my left shoulder is now sore.

Yesterday a onesie, which the British call a "baby-grow," arrived from England in a package addressed in Nick's mother's handwriting. It's light blue and white and made of a thick cotton jersey and terrycloth. Nick's mother even included the receipt and green plastic bag from Marks & Spencer, in case we want to return it when we get to London. She called last week to apologize about the color, saying she couldn't find any "normal" colors in the Marks & Spencer baby department anymore. But I was looking at the little card tied with a bow to the Pooh wrapping. It read, "To our new little boy, who we can't wait to meet, with so much love from Granny and Grandpa." They've been parents for forty-nine years, grandparents for nearly twenty. Unlike Mom, Dad, and me, they know what they're doing.

Nick's folks are traveling through France for the next three weeks. His father sent us the phone and fax numbers for every single place they're staying, except for the one in Toulouse, which doesn't have a phone. They've called each weekend for the past month to find out how we're getting along.

Worked with a migraine yesterday that only became bothersome in the middle of the night. So I took a pill. I've taken twenty in the past nine weeks, or roughly two per week, but my headaches are returning with the frequency they used to come, and I'm going to ask for a refill tomorrow. I've been doing well with very little medication. I suppose some women would have taken no medication unless they faced a life-threatening situation, but for me it's been a process of learning to increase my pain threshold. I'm proud that I've so far raised him on moderate quantities of good food, rest, exercise, and work. He seems strong and healthy at each checkup. I hope he's OK when he comes out.

Is it possible that I could love him already?

It doesn't seem possible that I could *not* love him. It hasn't struck me like a lightning bolt. It has accrued by doing simple things over and over for a long period of time, in the name of another person's well-being. Each day for the past eight months I've taken him into account when making nearly any decision. Step by step, bit by bit, I've come to love him — and I don't even know what he looks like, or who he is.

❦

Twelve days till due date. Five-thirty in the morning, and I've gotten only four and a half hours of sleep. Last night I started having contractions every fifteen to twenty minutes, some lasting one or two minutes. But I don't feel in my body that he's coming. Not today. The contractions harden everything in the lower part of my torso, making sleeping difficult, especially when they're so frequent.

What if he *does* come today? I'd be through with the process. I'd have to let go and let him come. No more anticipation. I'd be a mother, not just a pregnant woman.

I am waiting. There are many things I want to write, but I live outside of my mind increasingly these days, waiting for my body to go into action.

I want to write about how hard it has been this week to let go of my work. And trust that it will be there for me when I can return to it. I'm writing a story about welfare reform for the client newsletter. I've interviewed six of their staff and downloaded the state law from the web . . .

. . . Is it my imagination, or do I feel my cervix stretching?

Oh — I don't want to think about anything. I just want to sit and read, take slow walks, smell the early autumn air, and wait. It could be nearly another month.

On the other hand, I don't want anyone else to write this welfare story. I'm going to try to draft it today, along with finishing a couple of other jobs. It would be a disaster if he came today. Well — not a disaster; none of the clients needs their stuff right away. I could send some things off today and hand the rest over to Jeri. But I don't want to, control freak that I am.

I wish I could just record a message for my voice-mail that says, "I'm going to have a baby any day now; I'm out of the office indefinitely; at the sound of the tone, please hang up." I want to get ready to be totally taken up with our baby.

We thought maybe he'd be here by now. I momentarily suspected he might be coming—the contractions seemed to be taking on an action of their own. But they're only Braxton-Hicks contractions—the uterus warming up for the real event. They start and stop, and they haven't gotten any longer or stronger—unless I walk, and then I feel paralyzed below my waist and unable to stand up.

He's changed his position again. His bum's sticking out more in front. Maybe this is what they mean by "dropping" or "engaging." The books say the Braxton-Hicks contractions help the baby's head sink into my bony pelvis. So maybe my cervix is stretching after all.

Yesterday I finished two client jobs—five billable hours. With a couple of naps stuck in. The only time I feel I get any rest is in short half-hour naps snagged during the day. Nights just bring frustration and physical pain—the sharp pain of practice contractions that harden my belly until it feels like a strange, heavy ball, a separate weight laminated to the front of me, that stabs when I shift it. The pain of staying in one position for too long, circulation cut off; pain in my head, like a wasp buzzing and stinging. Pain in my lower belly when I stand up. It's hard to put up with. I think I've been pretty tough about it, but this morning, with my head having hurt all night and everything else stabbing me, I took a pill. Now I feel much better, but guilty. And worried. He's my son. Shouldn't I be able and willing to bear any amount of pain for his sake? I'm already a bad mother.

Bullshit. I have to take care of myself, too.

I've noticed that he now continues to move around even after I've taken a pill. He must be getting to be a big boy.

I'm so exhausted.

Nick dreamed that he came out, healthy and beautiful, and started to nurse right away.

꙳

I didn't realize until just before dozing off last night how much I was bothered by writing our wills yesterday. Our Quaker friend Zig, who is a lawyer, came over in the morning and helped us figure them out. Nick began to research what to leave to whom, and I thought my head was going to burst. Here I am in the extremity of pregnancy with our baby, and he's asking me matter-of-factly what I think should happen when he dies.

The baby rolls around in his cramped space. He no longer bounces, but he stretches his legs, and his fists continue to pummel my bladder.

Each time I pass his crib I wonder when he'll come. I wonder where he is on his journey.

My friend Jan said the other day that our baby is "still in that place we forget about after we're born." That he's in the process now of coming into the lifetime he's beginning, and forgetting the many that he's left behind. I love the things Jan says. They're so informed by her practice of yoga and Reiki, a kind of therapeutic touch that rebalances the body's energy. What she said resonates with the feeling I had in the month before I got pregnant, while reading Hillman's book about the daimon, of being hunted down by someone looking for me. This little person, in between worlds, looking for me — because he needs to know something I can teach him. And because he's going to teach me. He already is, and he's not even here yet.

"You guys are so *fucking* amazing!" our friend Johnny said yesterday.

"Why?" Nick asked.

"Because despite my cynical exterior, I'm an optimist at heart," he said. "Having a kid is one of the most optimistic things you could ever do. It shows faith in the future."

🖐

Nine days till due date. Nick is in the dining room holding a meeting of the committee that runs the London Program, the academic program that Nick will be teaching for in four months. He's now the committee chair. I baked them a batch of scones and they're in there having tea and laughing.

Put in three billable hours today. Feeling very lethargic — head hurt, still hurts, and I've taken nothing for it. This regression back to the chronic head pain I had before I got pregnant has to be a hormonal shift in preparation for labor. Something's happening with my hormones that I don't know about. With each passing day I feel more and more premenstrual.

Called a phone number for a "wicker baby basket" advertised in the paper. The woman on the phone sounded old. She said it was in good condition and had a mattress, and that I could come by to see it.

When I got there, the door was open, and I saw the basket sitting on her living room floor, amid a melée of junk. A yellow-straw basket with a hood. I had expected wicker—rattan—not straw. But it seemed sturdy and portable: he could sleep on the table while I cooked dinner, or on the porch floor while I paint, or on the grass while I garden. I could buy one of those mosquito nets and drape it over the top.

The woman came after I rang twice and banged on the door. She was old and stooped, with a frizz of iron-gray hair and blue eyes that sagged in her face. She wore pink polyester pants that hung loosely about her pouched-out waist. "Is a good basket," she said. "Baby can sleep in it."

The handles were broken. I began to imagine ways to fix them. I sniffed the foam mattress—his nose would rest against it, after all. It didn't smell bad.

"You know what you are expecting?" Before I could answer, she said, "You are expecting a boy, yes?"

"Yeah, I'm having a boy."

"That is what I say," she said, her mouth crinkling in a grin.

"How did you know?" I asked politely, figuring it would be the same old story.

"You are all in front, right here," she said, patting my basketball belly. "With boys, it is all right here. With girls—ugh!" She rolled her eyes.

"You know this from experience, huh?"

"Aye—with my daughter, I was sick all the time, I could not eat, I throw up all my food, I could do *nothing*. With my boy—*no* problems!" She cast up her hands. "You feel very good, yes?—you are having a boy."

"I hope I can be a good mom," I said, a bit distractedly, then decided I should just keep my mouth shut or pretty soon I'd be standing there bawling in her living room. I kept my eyes on the basket — I'd have to fix the handles; maybe I could find some leather thong and braid new ones.

"Oh yes — why not?" she demanded, her eyebrows drawing together severely. Because my brain echoes with the yells of an unhappy, trapped mother, I nearly said. A mother who through no plan of her own had two children within eleven months and no family or friends nearby (the doctor told her, after she had me, that she probably would never be able to get pregnant again, so she didn't bother to be careful); a woman whose intellect had been designed to derive fulfillment from challenges greater than — or at least in addition to — washing diapers, mashing bananas, and playing Weebles. Do they still make Weebles? — those little plastic egg-shaped people with weights in the bottom of the egg to make them stand back up when they toppled. "Weebles wobble but they don't fall down" — the seventies ad jingle. Judy had two families of Weebles, which she would pile into a Weebles Winnebago. "There were days," Mom always said — and her eyes would roll and her voice sigh with weariness when she said it — "when I'd think to myself, 'If I have to invent one more Weebles story . . .' " and her voice would trail off. The repetitive tasks — washing clothes, scrubbing floors, cooking food, bathing bodies, and her nemesis, ironing — gave our family a sense of coherence and being cared for. At the same time, they frustrated Mom no end, because they always needed to be redone. Undoubtedly, they've frustrated many women besides my mother. I'm sure they'll frustrate me: both Mom and I thrive on a sense of accomplishment, of bringing a job to closure. Whether it means I'll wind up yelling is, I guess, a question that only time will answer.

"Every woman wants to have happy, healthy baby—you, too," the old woman said. "You will be very fine."

I hope so.

The baby moved and the pin-tucks on my dress danced. I paid her and she held the door open for me.

"You have a name for baby?" she asked.

"Jonathan." We're not "telling" anyone, but now and then I figure it won't matter to tell a stranger. I like to run my tongue and my teeth over the name: Jonathan.

"Ah—Jonathan: is good name," she said.

As I hauled the basket and the baby across the street to the car, I noticed that, inside the car parked behind mine, a woman sat behind the wheel. She was watching me carry my baby bed back to my trunk. And smiling.

Nick has been meeting with the London Program instructors. One of them says her brain has been "offline" since her son was born three years ago, because she only took two months off work and then rushed to finish her book. When I described my timetable and told her it feels "too luxurious" to take seven months off work, she said, "I think you should take every luxury you can get."

She had three days' work left on her book when her son came. After he came, it took her months to finish that little bit.

I had my first daydream today that I could make my kid happy. I was singing and thinking about how he can hear me sing. I was thinking about how, after he comes out, he might be comforted when I sing. He might recognize my voice and remember his comfortable life in there, even if I don't sing baby songs all the time. "It's amazing how much they're comforted by your presence. It's an amazing power you discover you have," the London Program instructor said.

Sometimes I ask God to take care of me. God does take care of me, but not in ways that I decide to recognize or accept. It's like that old joke about the guy drowning in the flood, and he's sent a boat, a raft, and a helicopter, and he refuses them all because he's waiting for "God" to save him.

I *can* take seven months off. But *will* I?

At our visit to the midwives' today, we had Eileen Minnock, the Irish woman who had all her kids at home and delivered one of the other midwives' kids at home. She likes Britain's Radical Midwives. "They're *really* radical," she told us. "They *want* home birth."

I told her I was worried that my pelvis was too small. I looked at my chart today, really read through it for the first time, and the record from my first visit says it's "small-average."

"Do you think it is?" I asked.

She furrowed her brow and said, "Hmm, I don't know: how big are your feet?"

"My feet!" I said. Nick laughed. "A size 9."

"Pretty big," she said. "Your feet tend to be a good indicator of how big your bone structure is."

She examined me, and after all the contractions I'd been having for days, she said I was *still* only one centimeter dilated—"one good stretchy centimeter, and the cervix is well forward," she said encouragingly. "That's what all those contractions did for you. Good work!" I could tell she was humoring me. It was *only* one centimeter.

Her attitude was so practical. "I never measure a woman's pelvis till she's in labor. *Everything* changes by then, anyway—your bones spread, all the hormones loosen everything up. And if you measure at the beginning of pregnancy, then the woman's stuck with that image for months.

"And every labor is different," she emphasized. "I once had a woman whose baby wouldn't even move down into her pelvis—and the 'responsible' thing for the midwife to do in that situation is to prepare this woman for surgery. So I was all ready to say to her, 'You may have to prepare yourself for a section.' But in a couple of days she was back in, and she had an eight-pound baby in two hours. You can *never tell.*"

No measurement or other evidence, it seems, means anything at this point. Luisa is also one centimeter and 50 to 60 percent effaced, "but they said that doesn't mean anything," she said.

"It doesn't mean shit," said Judy, who is *also* one centimeter dilated. "We could walk around like this for the next three weeks."

We're all at the end of our rope. None of us is getting any sleep. Luisa and I talked about how our superstitions prey upon us. The babies look healthy during our checkups, but we still obsess over something drastic happening during labor. "You go in and everything's OK," Luisa said, "and then all it takes is to come out on the street and see someone with a problem, and you think the baby's going to be born with it. It's crazy."

Trying to lighten up about the whole thing, I downloaded a grinning mug shot of Martha Stewart and emailed it to Judy. She's a loyal Martha fan — or at least, a loyal fan of her recipes. I hope it makes her laugh.

The only reading I can concentrate on these days is Dr. Spock. *Baby and Child Care* was Mom's Bible, but I'm sure Spock has changed his views significantly in the last thirty years. In the edition Von and Dale gave us — the fiftieth-anniversary edition — Spock talks about playtime being a young child's primary way of learning about relationships. He urges parents to get kids together regularly with other kids beginning at two years old, three at the latest. I thought about how this means a good child care situation might be good for our baby. Joe and I sometimes saw our cousins on Sundays after church, but we never met any other kids on a regular basis until we went to first grade. I remember walking into that room and seeing twenty other children — a sea of other people all pint-sized like me — staring back at me. I want our baby to have friends as soon as he knows what the word *friend* means.

The midwife says he's at zero or minus-one station, and that he's "a good-sized baby," about seven and a half pounds. He's coming soon.

❦

I guess the Martha picture went over like a lead balloon . . .

Don't take it personally, but I don't really want to see a picture of Martha Stewart.

The itching has decreased a lot, but I generally feel like I've been in a bar fight and lost. I'm just about beyond my ability to be even barely civil to anyone.

I hope you're doing OK. I guess this is almost over, but I don't really believe it. I wish I could be sedated until I go to the hospital, but no such luck.

Take care.
Judy

🖐

He's coming. Woke with some hard pains that came out of my back, at about 3:30 or 4:00. That's the difference between these and the Braxton-Hicks contractions. These come out of the back. The Braxton-Hicks were only in the front. Another difference is, these aren't stopping. They're like fifteen minutes apart, but they keep coming and coming.

Just now I had some bloody show. That word again—*show*. Pink mucus from the cervix opening.

I was right after all. He's early by nearly a week. Yesterday morning I had a suspicion that he was coming—I was in the bank cashing a check, and I had to dash for the bathroom. In the bank. Everything let loose, with cramps, my body clearing itself out. "You're coming?" I asked him.

It echoed in the stall. "Is that what you're telling me—you're coming?" I had no appetite at all yesterday—everything just the way the midwives said it would happen, but still I could hardly believe it.

No more nights alone with Nick. No more passion. Here I am, at the end.

Here I am, at the beginning. Here comes another contraction, starting in my back, creeping around front, clamping down, turning my belly to steel.

And I'll get to see his face!

Half past ten in the morning now, and I'm taking a break from finishing some work—putting together a package on disk of everything Jeri might need; printing out Von's envelopes with her return address, as I'd promised. Leaving some last-minute phone messages. "You're *working?*" Nick said. What else am I going to do?—sit around and time each contraction? There are going to be *hundreds* of them. I have to do something to distract myself from the pain.

The midwife on call said it all looks like labor. But the weird thing is, you can never really know. The contractions are a lot like the practice ones. They don't come with a poster that reads, "You Are in Labor." In my body I know he's coming, but my head keeps questioning. I wonder how long it will be before I let my head turn off and I go into my body.

"It must not be long now," said the woman behind the counter at the Italian grocery yesterday. "A week from today," I said. "I was gonna *say*— you're really *low*, honey; Jee-zuss!" she said, staring at my huge belly.

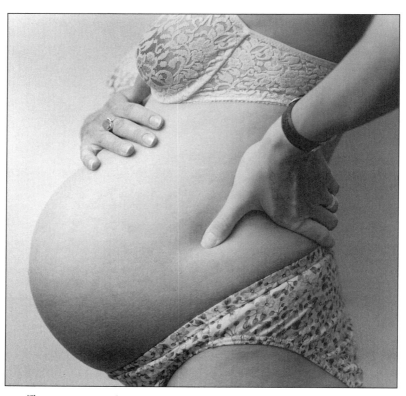

Thirty-seven weeks pregnant.

"Low." I would love to study the geometry of pregnancy. In fact, since he "dropped," I've been able to walk without my right leg cramping, and have been able to sit a full billable day at the computer without a searing backache. I asked the midwife about this. She said as the uterus grows, the angles of its drag on the spine constantly change. As his head has settled into the pelvic bones, he's relieved the pull on my abdominal muscles.

It's now 6. Half an hour ago I called Nan and told her we might have a baby by tonight. She started to cry, she was so happy, and I laughed. Then she stopped crying.

"How long have you been having contractions?" she asked.

"About twelve or thirteen hours."

"You have a long way to go," she said. "If you're able to laugh, you have a long way to go."

Postpartum

Our son was born two days ago.

We named him Jonathan Matthew. He was six pounds, thirteen ounces, nineteen and a half inches long. Beautiful, with clear skin and lucid, alert eyes of a stony blue-brown. A dimpled chin, just like Nick's.

We were in labor thirty-one hours. The pain was nearly beyond my endurance and I almost opted for an epidural. Anesthetic, true numbing out. But Nancy the Midwife, Megan the nurse, and Nick helped me through, and after more than two hours of pushing he was born at 10:15 A.M.

When they laid him on my belly and I saw his face, and his eyes opened, I forgot everything that had gone before, the tortuously slow progress and the *PAIN* of a strength and persistence that no one ever warns you about because they can't. Either they describe it and in your pregnant ignorance you don't hear, or they can't bring themselves to enlighten you so they just don't tell you.

"I had that experience with Carter," Von said on the phone that afternoon, "but I just couldn't tell you about it."

"That's the way it was for me," Nan said yesterday.

"With Sam?" I said. Sam is her elder son. They always say first childbirths are the hardest.

"With both Sam and Simon," she said. "But how can you tell someone about that during their pregnancy? They're already nervous and worried. It's important to have a happy, calm pregnancy: that way the baby's happy."

As our baby is, already.

I'm in love with him. I was right away. I'm surprised about that. Beforehand, I was worried (when am I ever not worried? — when will I ever learn worrying does no good?) that I wouldn't want to touch him until he was cleaned up. The idea of vernix and meconium grossed me out.

But when they put him on my belly, all covered in blood and mucus and some meconium, I couldn't keep my hands off him and I didn't want to let him go, and I was blown away by love. Like Nick said, it was the floodgates being raised.

Even now, at less than forty-eight hours, I hate leaving him for even a few minutes.

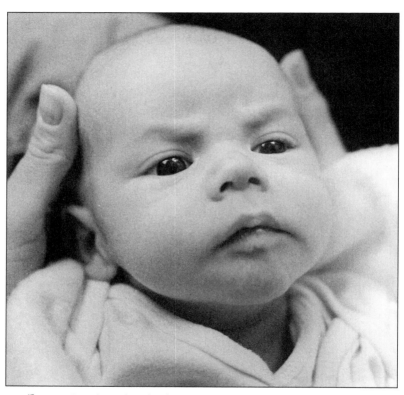

Five weeks after childbirth.

I have never, ever even wanted to risk feeling so attached to another person. What has happened to me? – I've become a mother, as though in spite of myself.

I want to write as much of it down as I can before I forget anything, even though I've got a terrible migraine and the last remnants of my sleep have been destroyed.

We came home the same day he was born. Von and Dale came to the birth center a couple of hours before we went home. Von was carrying a huge thing wrapped in a red bag from a toy shop. When she set it down on the floor I handed her the baby, and she just melted into the rocking chair and sat cooing to him for half an hour, while Dale stood beside her smiling and smiling.

Here I am calling him The Baby already. Like a mother.

Inside the bag were a red wagon with slatted wooden sides, and a pair of hiking boots made for a toddler. "This kid's gonna play, huh, Von?" I said. I couldn't believe she bought a wagon and boots. "He's going hiking with us at the cabin!" Von said. "Aren't you, pal?" Their visit felt to me like a benediction for us before going home.

Mom and Dad came to the house later. I had no idea how they'd react to seeing their first grandchild. They were tender and vulnerable and beautiful to watch, as though a layer of their skin had been peeled back, leaving their nerves exposed. As Dad held him in his big hands, I thought I saw his eyes go soft and wet. "Welcome to the world," he murmured.

Mom sat next to Dad and said to him, "Your mother would have said, 'He still remembers the angels.' "

❦

Here he is, five days old — not even, because it's only 7:45 A.M. — lying on our bed, hiccupping the way he used to inside me. When he hiccups, his whole little body jumps.

My love for him exhausts me and renews me. It's so powerful that it makes me afraid, as though I were being sucked down by an undertow too strong. Four or five times a day I cry helplessly in fear and love and bewilderment.

❦

Judy had her baby at 8:20 this morning. One day late — she went into labor on her due date, and had the baby on mine! Laura Elizabeth, nine pounds, one ounce. I have a niece! I cried on the phone when Judy told me, and she called me silly. But I'm so happy they're OK.

"I gave my love a baby/with no crying . . ."

Each day is a roller coaster of feelings. When he cries I feel all torn up inside, as though he's screaming at me in blame for bringing him into this painful world. All his little nerves are so raw. It was so dark and warm and comfortable where he came from. Why were babies designed such that they can cry before they can smile? I have spent the day talking to friends and lactation consultants and Nick and have come to the conclusion that he will scream and cry no matter what I do.

The ridiculous fact underlying my confusion is the image I had of a baby who wouldn't cry, or who would cry for a reason that he could tell me and I could fix.

The only way to get him to sleep without crying is to bring him into our bed with us and nurse him to sleep. This is difficult to do not because we don't want the baby in bed with us, but because we have a waterbed. It's waveless, but still, when Nick turns over, the baby goes flying.

Even now we're waiting for him to begin crying again.

Luisa's baby came today. I finally called the hospital information desk this morning. Yesterday I had stopped in on her at home, while out for a walk with Jonathan in the Snugli she gave us, and I found her in labor, lounging in a sweatsuit on the couch, trying to breathe and relax through contractions, hoping the painkiller they'd given her at the hospital wouldn't wear off before the four hours they said it would last. Her contractions felt strong to her but the hospital wouldn't give her a bed. They said she wasn't "ready" to have the baby. I don't know what I would have done if the midwives had told me I wasn't "ready" and sent me home when I arrived at 7:30 last Thursday night, after sixteen hours of labor. I was *ready*, even though it took fifteen more hours.

E.J. answered the phone and said it's a boy. "Soccer buddies, E.J.!" I said. He laughed. They named him Michael James. He was the same size as Jonathan and Luisa says he's "very cute." She sounded relieved that it was over. She's staying at the hospital for a couple of days. "I need to get my rest," she said.

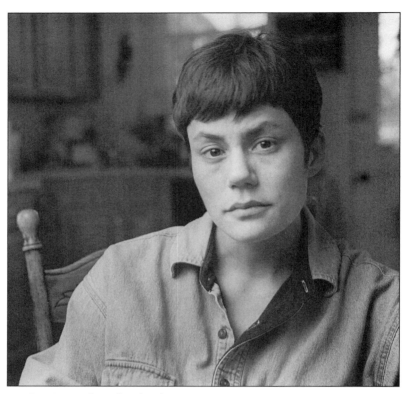

Six days after childbirth.

I don't want to forget about my labor. Emotionally, physically, spiritually, the hardest thing I've ever done in my life was have faith for a day and a half that something good could come of all that pain. I was in labor for thirty-one hours. Afterward, I felt that I could do anything in life. Meet any challenge.

That now seems a bit naive. The real labor is now. I am on demand constantly. No end in sight—he eats from my body. And gets gas. And cries. The other day I thought, quite naturally, "I feel so tired, I think I need a vacation. I'll just get away for a few days." Then it occurred to me that I'll never get away from this job.

I'm in tears daily, twice, three times, four. Sometimes I can't speak. And I wonder where my peace of mind went that I found when I was four or five months pregnant. It went wherever my sleep went. I can't sleep for startling awake, thinking I've heard him cry.

After a frustrating week of learning breastfeeding, bathing, and our baby's sleep patterns, I came home from our ten-day checkup with Nancy the Midwife yesterday in love with Jonathan all over again. My fears about his being colicky were relieved by Megan, our labor nurse, who handled him with the easy hands of a woman who has a baby at home herself. (She's pregnant with her second.) She sat in the office bouncing him on her lap, and he lay there, looking into her eyes as though he had a question for her on the tip of his tongue but couldn't get it out.

"He's wonderful," she said, with a starlit expression. "He's so *thoughtful.*"

Feeling better this morning than I have in days because Jonathan did not cry in the middle of the night. I nursed him at 1:00, he fell asleep at 2:30 without crying, and woke up again at 5:30. So I got two segments of unbroken sleep, three hours each. Plus a long nap in the evening. I feel almost myself and since he is sleeping in the sling on the front of me I want to try to write about the labor so I don't forget.

I managed yesterday to nurse Jonathan in a chair in front of Nancy's desk. Nancy asked me to talk about the labor. "Pretend I'm a cousin who wasn't here and doesn't know anything about it," she said.

Instead of a chronological memory of the labor, I had a string of jumbled impressions . . . the blast of fireworks from the baseball game at the stadium nearby . . . the helicopters landing at the hospital's trauma unit . . . someone saying, "Here comes the dawn," and looking out the window to see a faint pink light shining on the downtown skyscrapers. Most of the time, though, I was staring at a candle burning on the side bureau, while Nick supported my back or my legs. Nancy stayed at the foot of the bed with her eyes locked onto mine and gave me instructions: "Listen to me, Jennifer" or "You can do this, Jennifer." She squatted on the foot of the bed for more than two hours while I pushed. Afterward, her back hurt her so badly, she said, that she had to visit her chiropractor. But she wrote in my record that I pushed "very effectively, allowing for slow, controlled delivery of head." I had an intact perineum and only two stitches, she said, because I had followed her directions to breathe through many urges to push.

She says I had such a long labor because I'm not the kind of person who can surrender to her body without a struggle in her mind. "An intellectual type," she said, "and I can say that because I am, too, so it doesn't make it mean." She says she's had fifteen-year-old mothers hanging on her and letting her carry them into that uncontrolled place where the mind loses hold over events and lets the body do its work. Somehow, my mind held my body back for twenty-seven hours before letting go. I tried so many things — lying on my side, rocking on hands and knees, sitting cross-legged, standing in the shower, sitting on the toilet, hanging on Nick — but nothing helped me relax and give in to the contractions.

The pain was nearly unbearable. "Help me," I remember crying. "Help." I tried to think of the contractions as creative energy that was bringing my baby out. I tried to think of them as "rushes," the way the Spiritual Midwives do; I tried to think of my cervix as a flower, a lotus slowly opening its petals, the way I've read Indian women do. But my contractions were double-peaking and lasting more than two minutes, and I felt as though my body were splitting open. The contractions were not "rushes." I was not a lotus flower. If I was anything, I was a big beefsteak tomato, dropping from the vine, ready to explode its red flesh everywhere: I couldn't let that happen. For hours I tried deep breathing and "feather breathing" but nearly blacked out with hyper-ventilation, and I moved not by centimeters but by a millimeter here, a millimeter there.

Nancy proposed a narcotic analgesic. I had two shots, and for about an hour each, they took the edge off the knife ripping through my belly and relaxed my legs, which had been trembling uncontrollably for hours. But the contractions still wouldn't come any faster than four minutes apart. Finally, to hasten the contractions, she ruptured my membranes. I could not believe there was so much fluid. They had told me at my final prenatal visit that there were about two quarts in the amniotic sac. Kathy Evans-Palmisano had told us not to be afraid of squashing him during sex, that it would be "like trying to hit a Ping-Pong ball inside a water balloon," and I had looked at my tight belly in the last days and tried to figure out how it could contain two quarts of water along with seven pounds of baby. When Nancy slid in the white plastic hook and pricked the membrane, I expected a trickle of water but felt a warm gush spread down my legs and under my back. I sat up. The pads under me were full of water and blood. I'd thought that when my waters broke the pressure and pain would lift, but each contraction only bit more sharply and deeply into my belly: the shock absorber was gone. The lower half of my abdomen was trying to push him out, but my cervix wasn't cooperating. It wouldn't dilate beyond five and a half centimeters — only halfway.

At 6:30 or 7:00 in the morning, I crept on trembling legs into the shower for the third time, to try to relax. While I was in the shower, I found out later, Nick and Nancy were off talking about epidurals and hospitalization. I didn't know what to do to get the baby out. I asked for clearness — what Quakers call *discernment*. And standing in the misty bathroom, clutching the steel rail and struggling to breathe through the steam and the pain, I realized I would do whatever it took to feel our baby come into the world through my body. I didn't *decide* this, it was as though this knowledge came to me. It was *wei-wu-wei*. It was doing not-doing. I knew an epidural would cheat me out of that experience.

When I staggered out of the shower, here's what I knew: I had to not-do anything that would keep my body from doing its work. I had to not-try to dilate my cervix, because no amount of "feather breathing" or "creative visualization" was making it open. I had to get out of my body's way. I asked for another shot, to help my legs stop trembling and my mind stop clinging to the pain so it could step out of my body's path. In the next hour, my cervix dilated four centimeters.

I was in "transition." I could tell because I began to feel contractions that needed to bear down. My belly would harden like a rock, and the urge to bear down and expel the load was undeniable. "It wants to push," I gasped. Not "I want to push," but it does. My whole abdomen. But the opening was only nine and a half centimeters. It needed one more half centimeter, about three-sixteenths of an inch, before I was allowed to take a heaping gasp of air and push along with it. There I was, in that spot Sylvia had described in our childbirth class. Nancy ordered me to breathe through the contractions, but I'd wind up grunting and growling, "It wants to *push.*"

Then Nancy said she thought she could stretch my cervix that final half centimeter with her hand. I told her to go ahead. I felt her gloved hand slip inside me, then the stinging of my cervix stretching over his head: full dilation. I was so deep inside my body that I don't remember, but Nick said Nancy jumped up and down and clapped her hands. We were on the runway. The head was coming through.

It turned out to be a big head. Nancy says most babies' heads are twelve to thirteen inches around, but our baby's was fourteen. Nancy had me turn from side to side to keep the contractions coming fast and hard. I pushed with all my might—every three minutes, six to ten counts per push, five or six pushes per contraction—and I hadn't slept for a day and a half. "You're *excellent* at pushing!" Megan shouted. Words can't express how encouraged I was to hear this, even though I knew it anyway. Pushing was like finally having something to do after waiting forever. Pushing a baby out of one's body is, I imagine, like surfing: you gauge the speed and height of the comber, you work yourself into a certain position, you strain your entire body to maintain that position as you ride out the surf. Pushing was exercise. They had put a flannel robe on me after my shower; now I shed the robe, grasped my knees, and pushed.

"People aren't naked in the delivery room," a friend of mine had scoffed when I told her about the birth film. But after twenty-nine hours of labor and two hours of pushing I personified every scary aspect of the women in the film. Naked, bloody, sweaty, grunting, moaning, I was as unaware and as hyperaware as they were.

And like them, I just wanted to see the baby. In the film and in the books, they always tell laboring women, "The pain will help you see your baby sooner," and reading those books over the summer I couldn't imagine how seeing the baby would be an incentive for me. Getting the pain over with would be the incentive. But in labor, the incentive was to see the baby. The pain was the medium. I could feel his head boring through my hips. Megan kept monitoring his heart with the Doppler, and her touchpoint sank lower and lower below my navel.

"You see how far down he's come?" she'd say.

"I want to see his face," I would moan.

Finally he crowned. I felt as though I would split like the skin of an overripe peach. "You can touch his head," Nancy said. I put my fingertips to the soft-skinned roundness, and as I felt his hair I reached a second wind.

But his head got stuck behind my bones. For forty-five minutes, he'd come two steps forward with the push, and between contractions he'd slip one or two steps back. As the width of his head spanned my labia, I felt the exquisite sting of flesh tearing. My flesh. The sting was not at the bottom, in the perineum, but toward the top, near the urethra. I gasped, "Am I going to lose my clitoris?" I was serious. If having the baby "naturally" was going to mean losing my clitoris, then I was ready to say, "Let's just stop the whole show right here and wheel it into the OR." Nancy said I was going to be fine, but the stinging increased with each push—the rip tearing farther—making it harder to work with each contraction. I breathed and pushed, then waited—stinging and ripping—between contractions, and finally the pressure broke as, in the space of two pushes, his head was born. I felt it hanging heavy between my legs. Our baby was halfway into the world, partway in and partway out of me. I waited, savoring his pause before he departed forever from the tunnel he had made of me.

Nick stared open-mouthed at the space between my legs that I could not see as our baby's head hung there. Nancy asked for another push, and another, and one shoulder emerged. Then the rest of his body was born.

I've never felt such physical relief as in that moment. A friend with a daughter my age told me a month ago, "The birth itself is the perfect resolution to all that pain."

And here's the thing: when the nurse placed him on my belly, his back covered in a white receiving blanket, I could see his face, and I forgot about the pain. Fifteen minutes later she began to knead my belly to get my uterus to contract after the placenta came out. Nancy said my uterus had worked so hard for so long that it didn't have even one contraction of its own left; but it had to contract some more to prevent excessive bleeding. The nurse's hands felt like icepicks, and I thought, "I remember now—*this* is what went on for the last day and a half."

He lay crumpled, his eyes shut, utterly still, almost unearthly, as though he'd landed on my belly from some blue moon. I waited for him to begin breathing, but he just lay still, corpselike. Nancy says he was breathing the little tiny breaths that newborns take, but he looked so still. I could feel the cord stretching while the nurse suctioned his mouth and nostrils. To help him breathe, the nurse put a tiny clear-plastic oxygen mask against his face, quickly telling me and Nick, "This is *not* resuscitation." But he was taking some time to begin crying and we glanced at each other and at him, the panic palpable between us. Finally his little mouth opened into a rectangle and he began to cough, spitting phlegm. As I watched him trying to draw his first big breath, the first work of his life, I patted the crown of his head and held the mask to his nose and mouth.

Then he began to cry, and as he cried and cried his belly heaved against mine, and his face turned from blue to pink, like the sky over the city lit by the dawn three hours before.

Nancy handed the scissors to Nick, and he cut the cord.

And then our baby opened his eyes.

To think that I was afraid that Jonathan has colic. I just put him to sleep while rocking him in my office chair and reading my email. If he had colic, he'd never be sleeping like this. As I read the email posts in my in-box, he fell asleep at my breast. Now I can write, for who knows how long. I thought of Michele Murray's journal, which I used to torture myself with, thinking I could never work and be a mother at the same time: "For the past week [my son] has not slept at all unless he was rocked to sleep and even now I am rocking him with a foot and trying to write. I don't believe I've had more than two hours a day to myself (from 6 A.M. to 11 P.M.), and even those hours are divided up into fifteen-minute periods. I am a cauldron of seething frustration." Technology has made so many things possible since the day in August 1957 — forty years ago — that she wrote that passage.

Reading the birth record sent by the midwifery center, the feeling of immediate postpartum came back to me. Exhilaration with the success of having given birth and recovered so quickly. Thrill of seeing a new life begin its journey. The upwelling of love, so unexpected and different from any other love experienced.

And yet feeling empty. The liminality of the body emptied but still open. Watching the belly shrink, when it was so full and tight only hours, days before, and devoid of life when it had been jumping and rolling for months. Opened and leaking blood, water, tissue, when for months it had guarded and sealed within it another person, whole and healthy. The body soon to be thin and dry and cold again when it had spent months laden, warm with blood and water and life, working to grow another person. The breasts continue to grow, but the rest of the body lonely, cold and lonely. The back beginning to slouch out of loneliness: nothing to hold up anymore, nothing to work for.

And not even able to make love with my husband as comfort. Giving birth really is, as the midwife in Rothman's book said, a process of opening as wide as one possibly can. And I am still open. I am closing, but I am still open: the body in between states. At home, I am not allowed to take a bath. My cervix is still open, having stretched to its limit. My uterus is still healing, having sloughed off that temporary but all-powerful organ, the placenta. The only occasion in anyone's lifetime that the body spontaneously expels an entire organ. A self-surgery, an interior wound from which thousands of blood vessels must heal. Labia are swollen and perineal muscles bulging slightly from hours of skull-bone pressure during labor.

I miss the kicks. I miss the rolls. I miss the movement in the middle of the night that reassured me he was OK. I miss getting into the car and turning on the stereo and singing, knowing he will hear my voice in that swishing space of the uterus, the "storm" of the placenta rushing around him. I miss the constant companionship of him inside me. There is nothing like carrying another person inside your own body. He and I were both so restless that first night home that finally I lifted him out of his crib – where he looks so tiny and lonesome – and lay back down to sleep with him against my belly. He was quiet for the rest of the night, and I slept.

And to think I'd been so resentful of sharing that space with him. I don't wish him back there. I'm glad to be able to wash my feet without a struggle in the shower. But I still feel the loss of him from my body, the irrevocable separation of it. He is my son, but he and I will never be so close and harmonious again.

❦

He is sleeping in his basket. Who knows for how long.

I don't feel as though I will never write again. I feel as though I may not write for some weeks or months. I may just eat and sleep and take care of him for the next month or two. He's already nearly three weeks old. You hear it all the time, and it's true: kids do grow so fast. And as time passes he loses that crinkly, embryonic appearance. He looks less like ET and more like a little person.

Nick kissed my breast this morning and for the first time in weeks I felt heat between my legs. It was delicious. I can't wait until we finally make love. It's been months – since Maine. I haven't had an orgasm since *August.* And that one was the first in two months.

I will also enjoy getting on a bike. I might even enjoy the Nordic Track! I plan to express some milk (I can do it by hand, I've discovered — I don't have to use a machine) so I can get out for more than an hour without the baby. Or sleep for more than two hours.

I'm too tired to write. Consumed with his care and development. Feeling as though I should come up with something else to write about in here besides the baby, but he takes up all my days and nights, so why should I pretend that's not the case?

I'm as crazy in love with him as I have ever been with another person. All the fears I've anticipated these years about being a mother have not come to pass. I don't feel like smacking him when he screams. I don't feel like screaming back at him. I only want to help him. I have felt resentment, once several nights ago when he was up for three hours in the night, but I handed him to Nick and went downstairs for a break, and I was OK in twenty minutes. He cries, but not inconsolably, and I get tired trying to console him, but on the other side of that fatigue is that I *can*. With that ability comes satisfaction and intimacy. Here is this person who has so few ways of communicating, and I'm able to comfort him. I've found a way into his heart and mind.

Each discovery this kid makes is going to feel so exciting to me. Meanwhile, the ongoing daily care is so tiring. After he falls asleep, my mind feels unplugged. And my ears only want to listen to the silence.

Another two-day migraine, two and a half weeks after the last one. Maybe it's the lack of aerobic exercise. Maybe it was the argument Nick and I had yesterday. I went to the bakery at three in the afternoon when

Jonathan was asleep and apparently he woke up the minute I left and cried for forty minutes. And I said I'd be back in twenty. But it was literally the first time since he was born three weeks ago that I left the house alone, and I decided to stay out a few minutes longer. Nick held him clasped to his chest and threw me angry stares when I came back. He threatened to rent a cell phone.

"You can't do that to me," I said, bursting into tears for the fifth time today.

"*I* don't have a breast to comfort him," Nick said.

I'm in love with Jonathan, but my sole ambition is to sleep eight hours at a stretch.

Raising this kid is the hardest thing I've ever done. After the birth I said pushing him out into the world was the hardest thing. But it wasn't. The hardest thing is feeding him seven or eight or nine times a day for thirty minutes to an hour at a time. The hardest thing is staying in the house *all day* with nothing to do other than change his diapers, wash endless clothes covered with spitup and pee, and soothe his crying by walking him with my pinkie finger plugged in his mouth. (At least I discovered one thing that would stop his crying.) I swear he has telepathic powers that make him cry the moment I am about to do anything for myself—sleep, pee, bathe, eat, much less write or talk to another person on the phone.

But as I come to know him better, I'm more able to sense his needs and give him what he wants. Or at least I think I am. Last night, feeding him at 3 A.M., I realized the milk was coming too fast for him on the

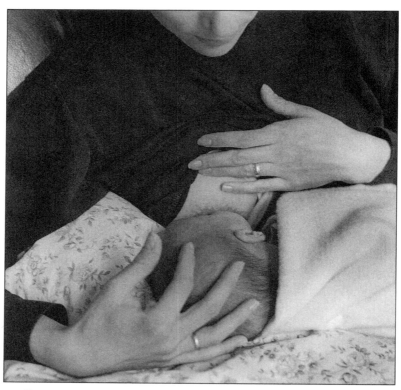

Five weeks after childbirth.

left then lay him down to nurse on the right so he could eat more slowly. And it worked.

Every day I ask myself at least a dozen times if I'm qualified to do this job. What qualifies me to be completely responsible for another person — and one so totally helpless and dependent? Sometimes I can't believe I wasn't required back in January to queue up in a line of pregnant women, where some regulatory authority would take a look at me and say, "OK — here's a list of reputable intensive courses in early childhood development; now pick one and sign up."

Jonathan is four weeks old today. It's 9:45 A.M. and he finally dropped off to sleep, after nursing for *an hour and a quarter.* Breastfeeding looks like the most passive job in the world, but it is such hard work. I never imagined it would be so demanding and intense. It burns up to eight hundred extra calories a day and requires me to sit still for up to nine hours out of twenty-four. (If I could have been that disciplined about sitting in front of my computer, I'd be rich.) Yesterday I felt at my wits' end because I nursed him for ninety minutes, part of it lying down, trying to get him to fall asleep, but he didn't shut his eyes for a second. I'm dying of fatigue and felt so hopeless about it after feeding him from 1:30 to 2:30 last night that I sat in the kitchen and ate chocolate frozen yogurt straight out of the carton.

The other side of it is that I'm crazy about him. All the love songs that play on the radio no longer apply to anyone but him. I sing them to him at the top of my voice, while he just sits in his vibrating seat on the kitchen table and turns his stone-colored eyes toward me. When I kiss his cheek he roots toward my lips like a baby bird, like he's giving Mummy a kiss, and it's the sweetest feeling I've ever felt.

I hope he likes me. He rarely looks me in the eye when he nurses. "It's probably still his most intense experience at this point," Nancy the Midwife said. He can't take more than one "stim" when he's nursing. Yesterday I broke down in tears after that ninety minutes of nursing and took him for a diaper change. I launched into a crying jag in front of him in the bathroom and accused him of not caring about me. And as I got honest with him for the first time, I think he actually *saw* me. He lay on the changing table and goggled his eyes at me and — I *think* — saw me.

What I learned from pregnancy to prepare me as a mother: go slowly. Trust my intuition, and trust my body. Eat regularly and moderately. Sleep. And all will be well.

So hard to follow all that advice and believe everything will be OK when the shit hits the fan — when, for example, the car's transmission has been diagnosed with a terminal illness and we have to buy another car.

Today I went to the dentist's office to have him fix a tooth I'd cracked last weekend. I was sure that he was going to tell me I needed a cap — at least one, possibly two or three, maybe a whole mouthful. But it only called for one filling, a small one, so small that the novocaine wore off in an hour. As he drilled, I had no trouble relaxing. When I was a kid I was so afraid of the dentist that I used to put a rosary in my pocket when I went (as though a rosary would actually *do* anything). Today I remembered the pain of labor and knew that nothing the dentist did to me could even come close. Go ahead, get out your pliers — make my day. The knowledge of my labor is in my body. It will always be there, the knowledge of my body's strength and endurance of the uncontrollable.

The only thing uncontrollable I think I couldn't endure is the loss of Jonathan. Yet my grandmother endured the loss of her second baby, a girl named Francie, when she was two. And that knowledge lived in her body and, together with losing her parents, two husbands, a house, and another middle-aged daughter, it made her know that a force wiser than she was in control of life and death — and teeth breaking, and cars' transmissions . . .

"I wish Grandma could know our kids," Judy told me this week over the phone.

"I think she does."

"Yeah — I think she's around, somewhere," Judy said, and her voice was soft.

So we'll get a new car, so what. Big deal.

Nothing is more important than the love that created this life and looks after it through doubt and fear.

We met little Laura yesterday at my brother Joe's annual October bonfire. Judy and I couldn't wait. "We'll have a baby-trading session," Judy had said over the phone from Cleveland.

It was so exciting. Right away, we handed each other our babies. Laura is so big — already twelve pounds, and Jonathan's still only seven and a half. "He's so *little!*" Judy cried. "Laura was *never* this little." She's beautiful, too, but in a different way from Jonathan. She has a full head of black hair, thick black eyebrows, and huge black eyes that tilt up and make her look as though she's smiling even when you can't see her mouth.

Already their personalities are so distinct. Laura is soft and cuddly and quiet. Even her head seems padded, while Jonathan's is bony. Laura clings to your shoulder and falls asleep; Jonathan is stiff, always upright, kicking and punching and looking around.

"He's like Joey was," Mom said.

She and Dad practically pounced on the baby when we set him, asleep in the car-seat, on the picnic table.

"I'll watch him," Dad said, towering over the seat.

"No, you go ahead and eat—*I'll* watch him," Mom said, hovering over the baby's face.

Maybe Mom couldn't imagine being a grandmother while the two of us were pregnant. Usually women become grandmothers with the birth of one baby; how many mothers have two daughters pregnant at the same time, and due within a day of each other?

For a lot of women, becoming "grandma" is a milestone that tells the world you're officially elderly, a fact of aging that cosmetic surgery cannot undo. But now that the babies are here, Mom's just reveling in them. She's falling in love with them. She carries pictures of them around with her everywhere. She has blossomed into a devoted, even besotted, grandma. I'm not sure whether she expected this, because it means being deluged with so many feelings, but it seems like she's really happy with the fact that she has two grandchildren.

I watch her hold Jonathan: she does that sway that mothers instinctively do — that I do myself, that maybe I learned from her — back and forth, her eyes half closed, humming or singing to him, patting his back or his bum. Calling him "Peanut" (everybody has their name for him: Von's is "Pickle," Jeri's is "Sweetie Buttons," ours is "Littley Man"). It's obviously a total-body pleasure for her, and probably is for him, too. At this point I don't trust too many people with him — I can't even begin to think about getting a babysitter — but I trust my mother completely, in an almost cellular way. Watching her take care of my son — with her careful and sure mother's hands, with all the movements and little sounds she learned in taking care of me and Joe and Judy — moves me and makes me feel closer to her than I have in years.

I remember when she was diagnosed with lung cancer, a little over three years ago. In the first threat of the word *cancer*, for a little while, the barriers came down between us and we could talk openly about our love for each other. Before she started chemotherapy, I went with her to four sessions with a wigmaker; after inviting her for six years to come to lunch with me in the city, she finally let me take her somewhere nice. She bought me flowers and called me "sweetheart." I remember saying to her, "Mom, you're going to get through this so you can see your grandchildren." I remember the look of surprise on her face when I said that — as though she hadn't considered that such a thing could be a possibility. Then, later, I heard her repeating this to other people: "Dammit, I'm going to see my grandchildren." Now, miraculously, she has two at once, and she's here to see them.

My having a child hasn't by a long shot fixed everything between us, but it has at least given us something in common. Now we're *both* mothers. It has given us something important, that we both care about, to discuss and dote on. To love.

🖐

Here I sit, on a Saturday morning, typing at the computer with Jonathan asleep in the sling on the front of me. It's almost like being pregnant again, I tell him, except now I can bend down and give him a kiss. The top of his head smells so good.

Three days ago, at my six-week postpartum checkup, Nancy the Midwife pronounced the process over. She examined the sites of the stitches and said they were healed. She palpated my pelvis from the outside and said she could no longer feel my uterus. The fundus, which was once fourteen inches high, jammed up under my ribcage, has now shrunk back below the line of my pelvic bones. My uterus sits right behind my pubic bone. It's so small.

I felt sad at the sight of her hand on my belly, looking for my uterus and not finding it. He used to live in there. My little boy. But he's no longer so little. The nurse weighed him as I was being examined, and he's eight pounds, eleven ounces now. No longer my tiny six-pound baby. No longer kicking up a storm inside me. He gets more and more used to the world every day, more and more independent. Each day I have to let go a little more.

But we are already close in other ways. When I undress him for our bath together, he might be screaming his head off until I pick him up and hold him against my skin. He quiets and clutches my chest and

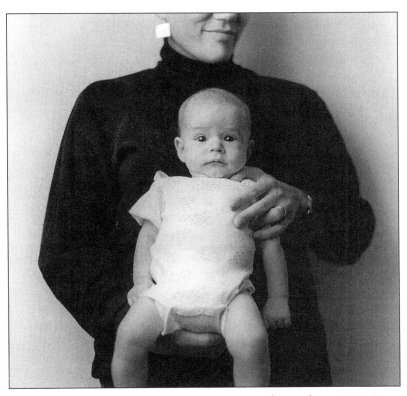

November 28, 1997.

arms like a monkey. ("We are monkeys," a Quaker friend who is a psychologist tells me. "I love that reflex. It's from our primate ancestors.") Then I step into the water, sit halfway and check its temperature as it flows between my legs, adjust it if necessary, and lower us both down into the warmth. I always remember the feeling of the warm water gushing out of me when Nancy ruptured my membranes. And then his face opens, like a flower under time-lapse photography, and as I hold him facing me on my thighs and swish water over his legs, he turns his wide gaze onto my face. His arms, his belly, his entire body relaxes: *Yes, I know where I am: I'm home,* he seems to be saying. I could swear it's a look of nostalgia on his face. He has never once cried in the bath.

We linger, reheating the water and floating and looking into each other's eyes. This week he began smiling, so I wait for his smiles and egg him on. When he's calm, I watch his face open and his arms and legs swish around, and I think of him floating in there, in the dark waters inside me, for nine months. He *lived* inside me, this little boy now curled and breathing the moist breath of earthly sleep against my chest. He lived in a space inside me that perhaps no one else, not even I, will ever see. Only he knows that mystery. As he sits with his legs against my flat belly in our bath, it's almost unimaginable that he was once on the other side of my skin, that he grew my uterus until it pressed against my ribcage, that he used to kick my bladder with such fierceness. Now my womb is back to the size of a pear. A *small* pear. It's closed again. And it's empty.

"I can no longer feel your uterus," Nancy said. She snapped off her gloves and said, "I officially pronounce you no longer pregnant." She told me I could begin any exercise regimen I wanted, that Nick and I could have sex ("Though most people are doing that before I even say those words," she said), and that we had to consider what kind of contraceptive we wanted to use because even though lactating women don't usually menstruate, ovulation could still happen and I could get pregnant.

Two weeks ago my discharge finally stopped. Then a week ago I began bleeding again, bright red this time, where the lochia had been straw-colored. Bright red bleeding in the first couple of weeks after it has been brown or straw-colored, the birth center handbook says, necessitates a call to the midwife. It might be a signal that part of the placenta is still in the uterus. It might signal a hemorrhage.

But it wasn't the first couple of weeks. It was five weeks. And I'd seen the placenta, the nurse showed it to me, and she'd said it was whole, she'd checked it. And I didn't feel weak, as though I were "losing blood." I waited a few days, and when it didn't go away I realized I was probably having my period. I haven't had my period since December of last year. In January, I remember, I prayed for it to come.

I told Nancy I thought I'd had my period. Her eyebrows shot up. You're not supposed to get your period while you're nursing full-time, all the books say so, and I certainly am nursing full-time, sometimes time-and-a-half when he just likes to suck. Jonathan nurses for at least forty-five minutes at a time, often for more than an hour, seven or eight times a day, with between-meal snacks. "It was bright red bleeding, and it lasted for five days, though it wasn't as heavy as a normal period. But I figure it was a period," I said, and she noted it in my chart.

"How many of your patients get their periods while they're nursing?" I asked.

She considered. "Less than 10 percent," she said.

I felt those old questions rise to my lips: *What's happening to me?* and, *Is it normal?*

"Why did I get mine, then?"

She shook her head at me in the same way she always does when I ask an unanswerable question. She opened her mouth to answer but I said, "Yeah, I know, no one knows, right?" No one knows why or how labor begins, no one knows how the placenta's hormone structure works, or how it coordinates such delicate communication with the pituitary, the corpus luteum. Nancy suggested we consider an IUD, because my vaginal muscles are not yet as toned as they used to be and won't be able to hold my diaphragm in place for another few months. I was reading about the IUD yesterday. The only one you can get in this country that doesn't have hormones is the "copper T," a little plastic T with copper filament wound around it. No one knows how an IUD prevents pregnancy, but it does more than 99 percent of the time. There's so much about this process that *no one knows,* that no one can fully articulate or explain.

As a matter of fact, Nick and I haven't been having sex. I remember thinking that after the baby came I was going to make love with Nick every day, and there have been many times that I've wanted to. But I've either felt too sore, or Jonathan wakes up, or we go so far and don't know what kind of contraceptive to use so we finish it some other way.

Which I guess is still "making love," but it's not the same. But then again, it might not be the same for a long time. Most of the time, we're just too damn tired. We haven't made love since we came back from Maine—more than two months ago. And before that my belly was so big it wasn't comfortable.

Now my belly is flat again. I've been doing the boring old Nordic Track three or four times a week, and after that I do boring old sit-ups.

I'm also a little afraid to have sex. I'm worried about how Nick will react to my body. I'm worried that all the "mothering hormones" will dry me up or make me leak milk, worried that Nick or I will find it disgusting or uncomfortable. Maybe I can't have an orgasm—who knows? I'm also worried about getting pregnant. I'm worried that Nick will see my body as a baby machine. It is a milk producer: I'm producing maybe a quart of milk a day for Jonathan, and he shows it, growing two pounds and four inches in a month. He drinks a *quart* of milk a day from my breasts—incredible.

They're big enough. Not as big as some other women's, for sure, but three times as big as they used to be. Nick likes them. This morning when I came out of the shower and he had just put Jonathan down for a nap, he knelt down and kissed them. It was immediate arousal for him. It's been *so long.* And he stood up and we kissed, and as we stood there tangled in each other my milk let down. I felt drips on my belly and legs. I pressed the palms of my hands against my nipples, anxious. "Oh, God," I said, "I'm leaking."

"So am I," Nick said, smiling. We laughed and jumped into bed. It was the same as before: we'd both forgotten to buy condoms, so we had to improvise. But it felt relaxing and restorative in the middle of so much hard work tending a small baby. His body felt new to me, newly strong and muscular, fragrant, and I buried my face in his chest hair.

He kept studying me, examining my skin and feeling the bones that had been embedded in flesh for so long. "Your body feels the same as it used to—but it also feels very different," he said. "Your belly's flat again, and your skin is still soft. But you also feel more open. It's as though you've opened your body to the widest, deepest experience you could ever have."

He ran his finger over my "linea nigra," the black line that winds from above my navel down to my pubic hair. The linea nigra showed up at about four or five months of pregnancy; it's the only mark pregnancy has left on my body, though many others have been inscribed on my heart and soul. One midwife told me she's hardly ever seen a pregnant woman with no stretch marks. Judy and Luisa might kill me for saying this, but as I get out of the shower and look at myself in the mirror I've sometimes regretted not having stretch marks, because I'm left with so little proof of the mystery of bearing Jonathan's life inside me. My linea nigra is the only mark on my body that gives evidence of my pregnancy.

"I love this line—I hope it doesn't go away," Nick said. "It's a sign of all the hard work you did. It says, 'This body once carried a baby.' "

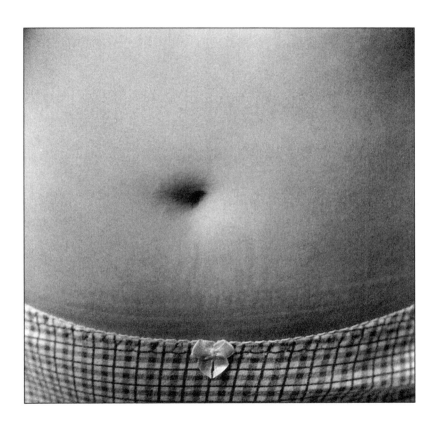

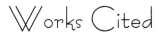

Works Cited

p. ix *Epigraph:* Kathleen Norris, *The Quotidian Mysteries: Laundry, Liturgy, and "Women's Work"* (New York: Paulist Press, 1998), 85–86. This exquisite tiny tome draws on Norris's poetry, her love of Benedictine tradition, and some deeply personal experiences to explore the mysterious ways in which commitment not to exotic or romantic life but to daily, *quotidian* life can open us to the deepest possible insights and transformation. This book also contains one of the few forthright acknowledgments I've ever read of the emotional, as well as the physical, rigors of pregnancy — "the psychic up-heaval, the bodily and psychic vulnerability" pregnancy brings (55).

p. xvii Jean Shinoda Bolen, M.D., *Crossing to Avalon: A Woman's Midlife Pilgrimage* (San Francisco: Harper San Francisco, 1994). This book brings together the experiences, scholarly discipline, ideas, and feelings of a woman at midlife. Throughout the book, the parallels between Bolen's physical journey to sacred sites (including Chartres and Glastonbury) and her consequent spiritual journey result in insights like this one about pregnancy.

p. vxii Terry Tempest Williams, *Refuge: An Unnatural History of Family and Place* (New York: Pantheon, 1991). In this book Williams uses her skills as a professional naturalist and writer, or storyteller, to take a close look at her location within several communities of which she is a part: her family; her Mormon faith community; and the community of wildlife at a bird sanctuary. The idea that "story binds us to community" is one that runs throughout the body of Williams's work.

p. 4 *Michele Murray's diary:* Michele Murray, "Creating Oneself from Scratch," in *The Writer on Her Work*, ed. Janet Sternburg (New York: W.W. Norton, 1980), 71–93. These moving extracts from Murray's personal journal, available only in this anthology, document her evolution from a 1950s newlywed to the mother of four children during the counterculture, and as a writer of poetry, fiction, essays, and book reviews. They span the years 1954 to 1974, when Murray died of breast cancer at the age of forty-one.

p. 19 *Kingsolver's collection of essays:* Barbara Kingsolver, *High Tide in Tucson: Essays from Now or Never* (New York: HarperCollins, 1995). Several essays in this collection about family, community, and the natural world offer a refreshingly honest and humorous look at how Kingsolver managed to integrate writing and motherhood, as well as her thoughts on why U.S. culture is less child-friendly than it could be.

p. 22 *The Millstone:* Margaret Drabble, *The Millstone* (New York: William Morrow, 1965). A comedy of errors, in which a single, twenty-something British career-academic finds herself pregnant after a one-night stand — and decides against the logic of her training to raise the baby. Remarkably, it was the only book-length story I found that explored (with keen insight into gender and culture, and deadly wit) both the anxieties and anticipations pregnant women face.

p. 32 *Estés's Wild Woman:* Clarissa Pinkola Estés, *Women Who Run with the Wolves: Myths and Stories of the Wild Woman Archetype* (New York: Ballantine, 1992). Draws on myths, legends, fairy tales, and other kinds of narrative, many from the author's own family, to offer women ways of expressing ourselves more authentically in our creative endeavors, spirituality, and relationships through reconnecting with our bodies and instincts — *"la criatura."*

p. 41 *dug out Adrienne Rich:* Adrienne Rich, *Of Woman Born: Motherhood and Experience and Institution* (New York: W.W. Norton, 1986; reissued 1995). Rich brings the language of a poet, the precision of a scholar, and her deeply conceived feminist perspective to bear upon her own experience of motherhood — her own narrative as it felt to her while she was having and raising her three boys, and how that experience was determined by and embedded within cultural ideas of "mother": what we are, what we do, and the cultural limitations we negotiate daily.

p. 49 *Roiphe's book on mothering:* Anne Roiphe, *Fruitful: A Real Mother in the Modern World* (Boston: Houghton Mifflin, 1996). Part memoir, part social criticism, amusing and streetwise, Roiphe reams late-twentieth-century feminism for failing to help women approach motherhood with more support — from male partners (passionately needed and loved by many women, yet repeatedly bashed by many feminists), quality day care, and their communities.

p. 54 *a Didion piece:* Joan Didion, "On Keeping a Notebook," from *Slouching Towards Bethlehem* (New York: Farrar, Straus & Giroux, 1970). In this essay Didion gives the clearest statements of the motivations for the creation of any piece of nonfiction: "I think we are well advised to keep on nodding terms with the people we used to be, whether we find them attractive company or not. Otherwise they turn up unannounced and surprise us, come hammering on the mind's door at 4 A.M. of a bad night and demand to know who deserted them, who betrayed them, who is going to make amends. . . . *Remember what it was to be me:* that is always the point."

p. 55 *that piece by Anne Tyler:* Anne Tyler, "Still Just Writing," in *The Writer on Her Work,* ed. Janet Sternburg (New York: W.W. Norton, 1980). A sweet essay in which Tyler relates, in anecdotes, the ways in which her writing processes intertwine with the ongoing processes of mothering.

p. 82 *Our Bodies, Ourselves:* The Boston Women's Health Book Collective, *The New Our Bodies, Ourselves: A Book by and for Women* (New York: Simon & Schuster, 1992, 1996). The progressive woman's health-care bible.

p. 104 *Julian of Norwich: Enfolded in Love: Daily Readings with Julian of Norwich,* trans. Sheila Upjohn (London: Darton, Longman and Todd Ltd., 1980, 1996). The divine visions of an English medieval nun who spent her entire life cloistered in a stone cell on the East Anglian marshes, and whose best-known "revelation" concerns spiritual surrender: "All shall be well, and all shall be well, and all manner of thing shall be well." The language of this translation from Julian's Old English is particularly poetic and musical.

p. 114 *Kathryn Rhett:* Kathryn Rhett, *Near Breathing: A Memoir of a Difficult Birth* (Pittsburgh: Duquesne University Press, 1996), 178. Rhett writes dramatically about the effects on her infant daughter of meconium aspiration—the experience, during labor, of the baby inhaling some of its initial fecal matter, which, for Rhett's baby, had life-threatening results.

p. 114 *Brazelton:* T. Berry Brazelton, *Touchpoints: Your Child's Emotional and Behavioral Development* (Reading, Mass.: Addison-Wesley, 1992). A wealth of observations and advice about children's development from birth to preschool, from one of the foremost American pediatricians.

p. 118 *Spiritual Midwifery:* Ina May Gaskin, *Spiritual Midwifery,* 3rd ed. (The Book Publishing Company, 1990). Written in the 1970s, this book is the classic reference on home birthing, compiled by a regular on the midwifery lecture circuit. In two sections: the first, telling stories in their own words of parents and midwives during the "natural childbirth" process at home (with candid black-and-white photographs of pregnant women); the second, a detailed technical manual for midwives (and also for obstetricians and nurses) that includes information on prenatal care and nutrition, labor, at-home birth, infant care, and breastfeeding.

p. 126 *Dr. Bradley's old-fashioned pregnancy book:* Robert A. Bradley, *Husband-Coached Childbirth* (New York: Harper & Row, 1965). The book that brought men into the delivery room, and the beginning of the "Bradley Way," one of the many methods of "natural" childbirth that emerged in the mid-twentieth century (others include Lamaze and Michel Odent's "Birth Without Violence"). Bradley's best-known (and most criticized) suggestion is that the father "coach" the mother by offering her instruction and advice during labor.

p. 168 *Rothman's book:* Barbara Katz Rothman, *In Labor: Women and Power in the Birthplace* (New York: W.W. Norton, 1982, 1991), 193–94. A well-written and well-argued study, by a feminist sociologist, of the history of maternity care and the medicalization and mechanization of pregnancy, childbirth, and breastfeeding in twentieth-century American culture. Interspersed with the author's own compelling accounts of her two "natural" pregnancies and labors, one a home birth.

p. 196 *Mitchell explains the Taoist practice of wei-wu-wei:* Stephen Mitchell, trans., *Tao te Ching: A New English Version* (New York: Harper & Row, 1988), viii. The best translation I've ever read of the eighty-one ancient Chinese poems, luminous with humor and wisdom, about how to live in accord with the Tao—the basic principle of the universe that to every activity, from good government, to child raising, business, sexual love, and ecology. Mitchell is a poet, born Jewish, has trained for decades in Zen Buddhism, and is a student of ancient languages and spiritual texts.

p. 200 *Hillman's book about the daimon:* James Hillman, *The Soul's Code: In Search of Character and Calling* (New York: Random House, 1996). A renowned psychologist argues that personal character and vocational calling are the result of one's "daimon"—"the particularity you feel to be you." Rather than encouraging individuals to see themselves as victims or results of their parents' practices, Hillman suggests that our "daimons" choose our parents before birth in order to learn particular lessons from them—and in order to teach them in kind.

p. 207 *Dr. Spock:* Benjamin Spock, M.D., and Michael B. Rothenberg, M.D., *Dr. Spock's Baby and Child Care,* 6th ed. (New York: Pocket Books, 1992). One of the most enduring pediatric references, Dr. Spock has lately garnered competition from pediatricians who argue for more "attachment-based" parenting, in which the child is kept physically near—or even on—at least one of the parents at all times (e.g., William Sears, M.D., and Martha Sears, R.N., *The Baby Book: Everything You Need to Know About Your Baby from Birth to Age Two* [New York: Little Brown, 1993]).

Acknowledgments

For a book such as this, in which the processes of writing and living are intertwined, it's important to me to thank those who contributed to both. I owe many thanks. To Judy Klatt and Luisa Bonavita, my companions in first-time pregnancy, as well as Dr. Timothy Klatt, M.D., and E. J. Bonavita III, all of whom generously agreed to let me represent their stories and our conversations. Judy and Luisa, you enriched without measure the writing of this book, and along with Laura, Elaine, Michael, and Christopher you continue to enrich my motherhood. To Charlee Brodsky, my collaborator and now my friend: "Our gardens will always be joined." To those who read the manuscript, in part or in entirety, and offered invaluable responses: Nancy Niemczyk, C.N.M.; Kathy McKain, C.N.M., M.S.N.; Evelyn Pierce; and Arsen Kashkashian.

To the following women for loving Jonathan for a few hours a day or a week to make it possible for me to write, and also for helping him to discover so early in life the meaning and value of friendship: Courtney Bradshaw, Nick's student who took such a shine to Jonathan in London; Katie Bartholomae, in Pittsburgh; Barb West, Michelle Ford, Marcy Bemben,

Lisa Henciak, Nina Randolph, and Marla Morrissey of the University Child Development Center at the University of Pittsburgh; and Pat Rabin and Carisa Weaver of The Right Place for Kids in Buffalo, N.Y.

To my editors at Crown: Linda Loewenthal, for her initial unabashed love for this project and Sarah Silbert, for her careful readings and for urging me to get brave and add dimension where much needed. To my agent, Gail Ross, for her hard work, love of good books, sense of humor, faith, everything.

To Nancy Abrams and Jane McCafferty, fellow writers, for their moral support and the gift of their optimism. To Von and Dale Keairns, for our Friendship, and for loving "our baby." To Jeri Spann, for teaching me the meaning of revision and for making me a part of The Team, and to Jeri and Evelyn for being Jonathan's Aunties. To Helen, for years of unconditional listening.

To Carmel and John Coles, for accepting me so immediately and completely into the big family that spans the sea.

To Joseph Matesa, Sr., for being so generous all my life and Jonathan's with his particular brand of patience and gentleness, and for understanding my need to write about my mother; and to Joe and Claudine Matesa, my brother and sister-in-law—along with Judy and Tim, my family of origin: "If I have not love, I am nothing."

To Nick and Jonathan, my family of choice. Nick, my dear Friend, thank you for finding me through the thicket of this world. Jonathan, my darling son, thank you for choosing me and for teaching me and learning with me every day.